AF443041

Imaging in Neurologic Rehabilitation

Imaging in Neurologic Rehabilitation

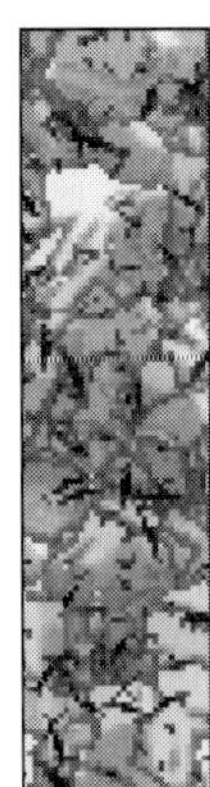

Edited by

JAMES F. TOOLE, M.D.

and

DAVID C. GOOD, M.D.

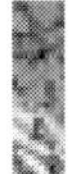

COMPREHENSIVE NEUROLOGIC REHABILITATION
VOLUME 9

demos vermande

Demos Vermande, 386 Park Avenue South, New York, New York 10016

Library of Congress Cataloging-in-Publication Data

Imaging in neurologic rehabilitation / edited by James F. Toole and
    David C. Good.
        p.   cm.— (Comprehensive neurologic rehabilitation ; v. 9)
    Includes bibliographical references and index.
    ISBN 0-939957-80-9 (hardcover)
    1. Brain—Imaging. 2. Brain—Diseases—Patients—Rehabilitation.
3. Brain damage—Imaging. 4. Cerebrovascular disease—Imaging.
I. Toole, James F., 1925–   . II. Good, David C., 1948–   .
III. Series.
    [DNLM: 1. Nervous System Diseases—rehabilitation. 2. Diagnostic
Imaging. W1 C04528 v.9 1996 / WL 141 I308 1996]
RC386.6.D52I38 1996
616.8'04754—dc20
DNLM/DLC
for Library of Congress   96-5287
                                                               CIP

Made in the United States of America

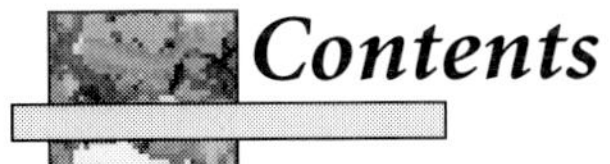# Contents

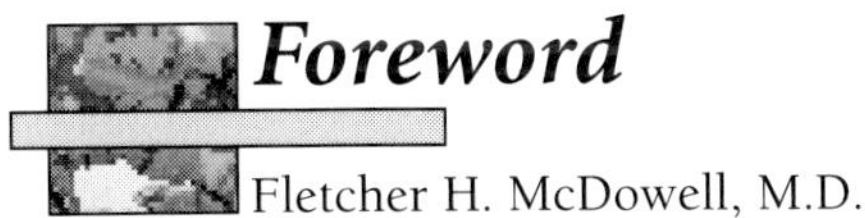

Foreword

Fletcher H. McDowell, M.D.

This volume brings together experts in the field of stroke research, and medical and surgical rehabilitation treatment with experts in the fields of neuroimaging, cerebral blood flow, and positron emission tomography, and explores ways in which recovery from neurologic illness causing physical disability can be tracked from onset to recovery and to discover how the central nervous system adjusts or reorganizes following injury.

Rehabilitation has a long history of being effective in reducing disability and, in some reports, reducing neurological impairments, suggesting a positive effect on neural reorganization and injury.

Until now, actual documentation of change in brain function has been impossible, but improvements in the ability of non-invasive brain imaging have made it possible to document anatomical changes as well as changes in function reflecting neurological recovery and its relation to improvement. The advances in neuroimaging have created possibilities for a more detailed study of the recovery of the areas of neural impairment and their relation to treatment. Rehabilitation treatment has in general been non-specific, but now it is possible to relate what is done in rehabilitation to specific changes in brain organization and function.

The needs for research in neurorehabilitation and rehabilitation in general are outlined by Drs. James Lieberman and Theodore Cole, who emphasize the need for documentation of changes in brain function and the effects on them of current rehabilitation techniques.

Drs. Roger Fiedler and Carl Granger report on the measures of assessment of outcome of patients following stroke and other neurologic illness. Their studies and development of the FIM scoring system have demonstrated the unique capacity of careful recording of function in tracking improvement in patients through the recovery and rehabilitation processes. Such information is of great importance if it can be carefully connected with the changes in brain function produced by imaging.

Dr. James Prichard outlines the use of magnetic resonance imaging techniques and the study of rehabilitation medicine. Advances in this field have been extraordinary. Not only is it possible to accurately identify actual anatomical changes in brain structure, but also it is now possible with alterations in MRI technique to image in real time accurate pictures of the cerebral circulation. Development of the echo-planar gene techniques have speeded up the process of magnetic resonance imaging of the brain, which can be done in milliseconds

The develop of magnetic resonance spectroscopy now makes it possible to determine changes in the metabolism during cerebral infarction of a large number of metabolites including high energy phosphates and lactate, which are essential for normal neurologic function. These are altered in tissue damaged by stroke, and the potential now exists for having second-by-second determinations of the changes in glucose utilization, levels of high-energy phosphate, changes in neurotransmitter release in the area of infarcted tissue and the surrounding impaired, but not dead, neural structures.

Dr. K. M. A. Welch discusses the potential of diffusion and T_2 MRI imaging. This makes it possible to follow the diffusion of water into damaged nervous tissue. It is possible to show the development of cerebral edema in an infarct and to distinguish between necrotic tissue and tissue that is functionally impaired but viable. Images in animal experiments with cerebral infarcts show clear delineation between the central infarct and the surrounding penumbra of viable tissue. He believes it is now possible to immediately distinguish the regions of necrosis from less involved tissue in areas of subacute ischemia. This may make it possible to rapidly identify the effects of neuro-protective agents that are being tried in treatment of acute stroke. Using these techniques could make it possible to clearly define the time of the therapeutic window in acute stroke where neural damage can be reversed or limited.

Dr. Sid Gilman reviews the potential of positron emission tomography in the study of changes in brain function following stroke, pointing out that it is possible to identify localized areas of change in metabolism of glucose, metabolites, neurotransmitters and neurotransmitter receptors in involved areas of stroke. Now it is possible to use PET scanning to study alterations and reorganization of brain function during recovery from stroke. Using PET scanning there is growing evidence that following a stroke in one hemisphere there are compensation changes in function in the opposite hemisphere and that these are possibly related to the improvement in function following stroke. These techniques are being rapidly explored in both the United States and Great Britain to enlarge the evidence relating changes of altered sites of brain function taking place following stroke to recovery and their relation to the process of rehabilitation treatment.

Single photon emission computed tomography is reviewed by John Keyes, who points out the ability of this technique to trace conventional radionuclides to study cerebral blood flow and changes in cerebral metabolism following stroke. Precise changes in blood flow and blood volume can be determined using this technique. In a report by Henrik Jorgensen and Niels Lassen using SPECT techniques to study spontaneous reperfusion following stroke was closely related to good outcome. This type of study could be used to allow a better determination of prognosis and the chance of a favorable outcome with rehabilitation treatment.

Studying glucose metabolism with PET during the performance of specific tasks and the relation of changes in metabolism in the human central nervous system has made it possible with real time analysis to localize areas of the central nervous system related to specific tasks and the psychological state of individuals being tested. This will allow better definition of cortical areas involved in motor activity and make it possible to track changes during recovery from stroke and head injury.

The role of pharmacotherapy in promoting recovery in function is reviewed by Dr. Dennis Feeney and Dr. Larry Goldstein. Both pointed out the major advances in this area using adrenergic agents in promoting recovery7 from both experimental stroke and head injury. These experiments have revealed a number of pharmacologic agents that can enhance recovery or impair it. An important finding in these studies was that recovery could be enhanced not only by pharmacologic agents but also by training and experience in task performance. This finding further supports the usefulness of rehabilitation techniques in restoring function and possibly in improving neurological function and promoting reorganization of cortical function following brain injury. Treatment of stroke with adrenergic agents following stroke has provided some early evidence that these agents may have a role in treatment of patients in rehabilitation following stroke. Clinical studies have provided preliminary evidence that some of the commonly used agents for sedation, blood pressure control, and relief of anxiety may have a harmful effect on stroke recovery. These are extremely important areas of research, as they have demonstrated the possibility to enhance rehabilitative efforts and have the promise of producing improvement in individuals with stroke.

Demonstration of widespread changes in neurotransmitter function in many areas of the brain other than the primary area of damage have enlarged the concept of what disrupted general neurotransmitter function can do in the way of impairing central nervous system function and how this may be altered with treatment.

Drs. Donald Stein and Robin Roof review the alterations in nervous system metabolism which can be potentially destructive events and can further impair neural function following damage with stroke or trauma. They reviewed the suggestions for preventing these inherent serious tissue damaging effects by current treatment. This is an important area relating to neural protective treatments that are now being evaluated in a number of centers. Better understanding of the mechanisms involved in neural injury following trauma and their role in repair following brain injury is becoming increasingly important.

Dr. Edward Taub and colleagues report on studies of improvement in function in an impaired extremity following stroke using motor restriction of the unimpaired extremity. They showed that forced use of a partially impaired extremity following stroke can result in some recovery of function. Combining forced use treatment with PET imaging of the changes in cortical function with this treatment has the promise of better understanding how rehabilitation techniques produce improvement in function.

The problem of speech impairment and reading problems following stroke is reviewed by Dr. Branch Coslett, who presents new strategies that improve cognitive processing and reading which may have great importance in helping individuals who have had brain damage that specifically affects their ability to read and possibly this may be expanded to the problem of difficulty speaking.

This volume demonstrates the possibility that investigations of acute stroke and head injury using current and future advances in neuroimaging will undoubtedly lead to a much better understanding of the rehabilitation process and what can be done to make it better and more specific and how this can be influenced by pharmacologic treatment. Now for the first time it is possible to connect rehabilitation with changes in brain function and physiology

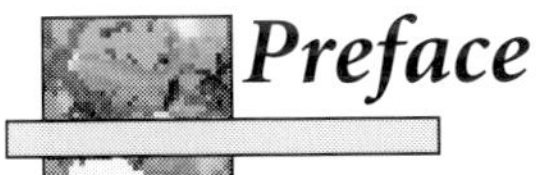

Preface

Functional neuroimaging techniques can provide a minimally invasive and quantitative scientific way to investigate the functioning of local areas of the brain and spinal cord by direct measurement in the living patient. Research studies over the past two decades using positron emission tomography (PET) have demonstrated the sensitivity of functional imaging in detecting abnormalities of the brain related to aging, dementia, tumors, seizures, dyslexia, cerebral vascular accidents, and psychiatric problems, amongst others. Important results also have been reported by investigators using other imaging modalities such as transcranial Doppler imaging (TCD), magnetic resonance imaging (MRI)* and magnetic resonance spectroscopy (MRS), computerized tomography (CT) (especially in image fusion with PET and SPECT), single photon emission tomography (SPECT). magnetoencephalography (MEG), and electroencephalography with mapping (EEG). (1)

The important role of functional imaging in rehabilitation research using a multidisciplinary research approach is apparent in the *Goals and Research Opportunities* of the Research Plan of the National Center for Medical Rehabilitation Research, but until now research typically has progressed as disparate activities in a variety of institutional departments. All disciplines need a better understanding of the capabilities of functional neuroimaging as related to important unsolved problems in rehabilitation research in order to facilitate their eventual clinical application.

For these reasons, a three-day scientific workshop was held under the auspices of the Bowman Gray School of Medicine of Wake Forest University on March 11–13, 1994, in Winston-Salem, North Carolina.

The workshop was planned and conducted by an Organizing Committee co-chaired by neurologist Dr. James Toole and radiologist Dr. John Keyes. The Committee was comprised of experts in functional neuroimaging, medical rehabilitation research, neuroscience, and workshop planning. The Committee planned the scientific program and selected speakers appropriate to the general and specific workshop objectives.

The objectives of the workshop were to:

- Inform medical rehabilitation researchers about the capabilities of functional imaging.
- Inform imaging researchers about problems in medical rehabilitation research where functional neuroimaging may contribute to solutions;
- Engender continuing interactions between researchers in medical rehabilitation, functional imaging, and neuroscience, and foster the development of multidisciplinary research activities.

---

* MRI is inclusive term for medical imaging with NMR.

The scientific program was designed to focus on the impact of functional neuroimaging on high priority areas described in the NCMRR Research Plan (2). The format included presentations and structured discussion by experts in functional neuroimaging and medical rehabilitation research which addressed four of the vital roles of functional neuroimaging; generating basic scientific knowledge of brain function indices related to specific disabilities; locating the foci in the brain, spinal cord, and/or the peripheral nervous system; monitoring the temporal changes of lesions and of their clinical expression; and measuring the outcomes and effectiveness of surgical, pharmacological, and medical rehabilitation interventions.

These proceedings will provide valuable guidance about the contributions of functional neuroimaging techniques to the generation of the new knowledge needed ion developing a sound scientific basis for the field of medical rehabilitation research. The report also will provide valuable insight for the development of multidisciplinary projects in medical rehabilitation research.

We thank Mr. Gil Devey, Dianne C. Vernon, and Louis Quatrano who spearheaded this endeavor, Sara Ferner who transcribed the tapes, Pam Beck who prepared it for publication, and Dr. Diana M. Schneider who did the desk editing in preparation for its publication.

James F. Toole, M.D.
Principal Investigator
Director, Stroke Research Center
Bowman Gray School of Medicine

David Good, M.D.
Consultant
Director of Rehabilitation
Bowman Gray School of Medicine

References

1. Medline Search May 6, 1992, 1988 foreword. Key words: regional cerebral blood flow (243 titles); functional brain imaging (17 titles); receptor imaging (39 titles); brain radionuclide imaging (457 titles); brain mapping (58 titles).
2. DRAFT Report and Research Plan for the National Center for Medical Rehabilitation Research. National Advisory Board on Medical Rehabilitation Research, National Institute of Child Health and Human Development, National Institutes of Health. February 6, 1992.

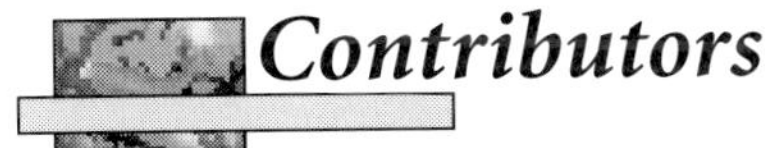# Contributors

Floyd E. Bloom, M.D., Biomagnetic Laboratories, Scripps Clinic and Research Foundation, 10666 North Torrey Pines Road, La Jolla, CA 92037.

Theodore M. Cole, M.D., Department of Physical Medicine and Rehabilitation, University of Michigan Medical Center, 1500 East Medical Center Drive, Ann Arbor, MI 48109-0042.

H. Branch Coslett, M.D., Department of Neurology, Temple University Hospital, 3401 N. Broad Street, Philadelphia, PA.

Jean E. Crago, M.S., P.T., Department of Physical Therapy, University of Alabama at Birmingham, Birmingham, AL 35294

Stephanie C. DeLuca, B.A., Department of Psychology, University of Alabama at Birmingham, Birmingham, AL 35294

Dennis M. Feeney, Ph.D., Department of Psychology, Logan Hall, The University of New Mexico, Albuquerque, NM 87131-1161.

Roger C. Fiedler, Ph.D., Uniform Data System for Medical Rehabilitation, 232 Parker Hall, SUNY South Campus, 3435 Main Street, Buffalo, NY 14214-3007.

R.S.J. Frackowiak, MRC Cyclotron Unit, Hammersmith Hospital, Du Cane Road, London W12 0HS, England.

Christopher C. Gallen, M.D., Ph.D., Biomagnetic Laboratories, Scripps Clinic and Research Foundation, 10666 North Torrey Pines Road, La Jolla, CA 92037.

Amy Garrett, Department of Neuropsychology, Bowman Gray School of Medicine, Medical Center Boulevard, Winston-Salem, NC 27157.

Sid Gilman, M.D., University of Michigan, Department of Neurology, Taubman Center 1914/0316, 1500 East Medical Center Drive, Ann Arbor, MI 48109-0316.

Larry B. Goldstein, M.D., Assistant Professor of Medicine (Neurology), Duke University Medical Center, Box 3651, Durham, NC 27710.

Carl V. Granger, M.D., Uniform Data System for Medical Rehabilitation, 232 Parker Hall, SUNY South Campus, 3435 Main Street, Buffalo, NY 14214-3007.

Yasuhiro Hasegawa, M.D., Division of Cerebrovascular Disease, Research Institute, National Cardiovascular Center, 5-7-1, Fujishiodai Suita, Osaka 565, Japan.

Henrik Stig Jørgensen, M.D., Department of Neurology, Bispebjerg Hospital, DK-2400 Copenhagen, Denmark.

John W. Keyes, Jr., M.D., Bowman Gray/Baptist Hospital, Department of Radiology, Medical Center Boulevard, Winston-Salem, NC 27157-1088.

Niels Alexander Lassen, M.D., Ph.D., Department of Clinical Physiology, Bispebjerg Hospital, Bispebjerg Bakke 23, DK-2400 Copenhagen NV, Denmark.

James S. Lieberman, M.D., Department of Physical Medicine and Rehabilitation, Columbia University College of Physicians and Surgeons, 710 West 168th Street, New York, NY 10032.

Hirofumi Nakayama, M.D., Ph.D., Department of Clinical Physiology, Bispebjerg Hospital, Bispebjerg Bakke 23, DK-2400 Copenhagen NV, Denmark.

Tom Skyhøj Olsen, M.D., Ph.D., Department of Neurology, Bispebjerg Hospital, DK-2400 Copenhagen, Denmark.

Rama D. Pidikiti, M.D., Department of Physical Medicine, University of Alabama at Birmingham, Birmingham, AL 35294

James W. Prichard, M.D., Department of Neurology, Yale University School of Medicine, 333 Cedar Street, New Haven, CT 06510.

Robin L. Roof, Ph.D., Department of Psychology, Texas Christian University, Fort Worth, TX 76129.

Barry J. Schwartz, Ph.D., Biomagnetic Laboratories, Scripps Clinic and Research Foundation, 10666 North Torrey Pines Road, La Jolla, CA 92037.

Bjørn Sperling, M.D., Department of Neurology, Bispebjerg Hospital, Bispebjerg Bakke 23, DK-2400, Denmark.

Donald Stein, M.D., Graduate School of Arts and Sciences, 202 Administration Building, Emory University, Atlanta, GA 30322.

Edward Taub, Ph.D., Department of Psychology, 201 Campbell Hall, University of Alabama at Birmingham, Birmingham, AL 35294.

K.M.A. Welch, M.D., Department of Neurology, Henry Ford Hospital, 2799 W. Grand Boulevard, Detroit, MI 48202.

John Whyte, M.D., Ph.D., Moss Rehabilitation Research Institute, 1200 West Tabor Road, Philadelphia, PA 19141-3099.

Frank Wood, M.D., Department of Neuropsychology, Bowman Gray School of Medicine, Medical Center Boulevard, Winston-Salem, NC 27157.

Tony T. Yang, M.D., Ph.D., Biomagnetic Laboratories, Scripps Clinic and Research Foundation, 10666 North Torrey Pines Road, La Jolla, CA 92037.

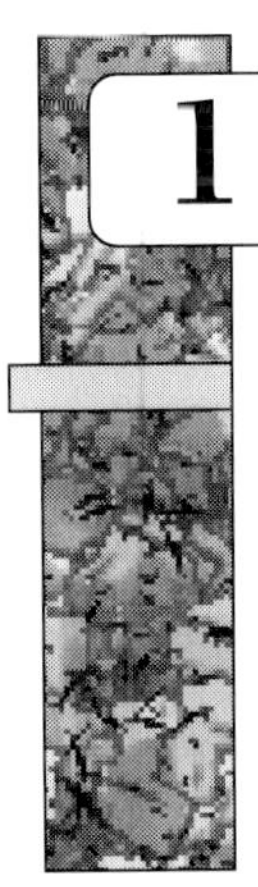

Introduction and Review of Mechanisms of Functional Recovery

John Whyte, M.D.

In order to evaluate the role of functional neuroimaging in rehabilitiation research, it is important to consider a number of potential mechanisms of functional recovery; to give an overview of some of the proposed models of functional recovery that have appeared in the literature; to explore their possible relevance in terms of clinical rehabilitation; and to examine aspects of these mechanisms that might be suitable for clarification by neuroimaging. This last point relates to whether one is talking about neurologic recovery or functional recovery; functional imaging technologies are more suitable for examining neurologic recovery. Functional recovery means recovery in the sense of success in acting upon the environment. Clearly, one can accomplish a task such as getting from here to there in one hundred different ways that might work quite well but which use different muscle groups, perhaps even different pieces of equipment or appliances. There is no reason to imagine that PET images of the brain are going to look anything alike if one is ambulating, crawling, or getting somewhere by wheelchair. This illustrates how different in some ways the ultimate concern of rehabilitation is from the concern of more basic science orientations or even, in many ways, neurology. Rehabilitation is interested in success in terms of *environmental outcomes*.

To point out more clearly the frequent mismatch between these two levels of analysis: it is possible to have good neurologic recovery within a particular domain and yet have a poor functional outcome. One example is a patient with traumatic brain injury who has paralysis and ataxia. The patient might show good recovery to normal levels of strength, yet be completely unable to accomplish a wide variety of physical tasks because of the remaining ataxia. Conversely, it is possible to influence functional recovery without impacting the underlying neurologic recovery. For example, pharmacologic management of urinary incontinence improves continence without repairing the underlying lesion in the spinal cord or brain.

1

A number of authors have discussed and reviewed proposed mechanisms of functional recovery. Some authors use slightly different terminology but the following basic breakdown is useful.

- Resolution of temporary factors refers to a variety of things that occur in the very acute period, such as resolution of edema, reestablishment of adequate circulation and oxygenation, and so on. Essentially these may have caused tissue dysfunction but not tissue death, and therefore there is a potential interval to intervene and salvage remaining viable tissue.
- Structural reorganization applies to dendritic and axonal branching and sprouting, meaning the actual establishment of some form of new neural connection as a response to injury.
- Unmasking or redundancy refer to changes in neural function that appear to occur too rapidly to be accounted for by mechanisms that involve regrowth or any major chemical changes, but which suggest the presence of connections in a latent form that are available for use.
- Neurochemical alteration refers to not only dysfunctional changes occurring acutely, which are probably responsible for many aspects of diaschisis, but also to the mechanisms that involve recalibration of receptors' sensitivities and neurochemical synthesis, which may allow less viable neural tissue to accomplish the same levels of activity after these changes have taken place.
- Vicarious functioning and functional substitution are in many instances difficult to disentangle. From a semantic standpoint, vicarious functioning is generally meant to indicate that not only does a new area of brain subserve a function but that it does so in some sense by altering its characteristics to become good at that function. Functional substitution more often means that a part of the brain that is good at one thing finds a way to accomplish this task using those same behavioral propensities. These are hard to disentangle because the better functional substitution works (that is, the more smoothly and capably a new neural system executes a task), the harder it is to detect the substituted strategy and therefore the more difficult it is to separate it from vicarious functioning.

Current therapy aims only at the top and the bottom of this list. The acute neurosurgical and neurologic care period certainly does what it can to minimize the influence of the temporary factors in causing further destruction. All of the teaching technologies that we make use of in rehabilitation care focus on the bottom end, that is, training people in alternate strategies, providing equipment and devices that allow for tasks to be accomplished by alternate means, and so on. However, we have very little in the way of rational treatment aimed at the other mechanisms.

We are probably the closest to having some rational intervention in the area of neurochemical alteration, in that we are rapidly learning about chemical modulations that can be influenced by drug intervention. Prior research strategies to look at mechanisms of recovery have included a variety of approaches: lesion studies (natural and induced; single and sequential) to look at what parts of the brain were able to take over function; histochemical studies; pharmacologic interventions in animal models; and psychological and behavioral analyses in which one infers the nature of the recovery in part by looking at the pattern of errors or the pattern of performance following recovery of function.

The animal literature on recovery of function has many of the same limitations that we have talked about in the neuroimaging domain. It has been easy to show that things change in the nervous system after injury, but it has been much harder to determine the causal relationship between those changes and the behavioral recovery that takes place. We are hearing the same things in terms of neuroimaging patterns post-injury, but it is still unclear exactly how to interpret their role in the behavioral adaptation, which is ultimately our interest.

The challenge was and remains to show that these particular changes are causally responsible for behavioral recovery. We also need to correlate the biological and psychological changes that we find (whether in histochemical or neurologic indices or in imaging studies) with various kinds of behavior.

In human neuropsychological assessment, one learns about recovery mechanisms not only by observing success or failure at a task, but also by observing the *process* and *strategy* by which the task is or is not accomplished. Interpretation of animal recovery literature has been limited to some degree by inadequate attention to task process and strategy.

There is a body of literature on motor recovery in animals that uses, for example, a task such as crossing a balance beam as an index of recovery. It allows one to look at gross recovery, but it does not answer the question of whether the muscle groups that used to be subserving ambulation are the ones now being used on the balance beam. For a more detailed understanding of how that animal recovers following a motor cortex lesion, one needs to know not just outcome—that they got from one side of the beam to the other—but the motor patterns involved, and the strategy or process that was used for accomplishing that task. The more we can take a detailed look at the process of task accomplishment, as well as simply success or failure, the more we will be able to link behavioral adaptations to underlying neural mechanisms.

What is the role of functional neuroimaging? We need to ask how neuroimaging approaches can distinguish among and clarify the roles of these different mechanisms at different points in time, presumably from the standpoint of clinical recovery. We are probably dealing with a messy blend of different recovery mechanisms that may overlap in time, and some of which may have dysfunctional outcomes. We need to use various analytic techniques to disentangle which mechanisms are responsible at which phases for which aspects of the recovery process.

We will eventually need imaging methods that can track performance of more complex tasks. Ultimately, the functions we are interested in are far more complicated than finger tapping, and we need to find some way to bridge the gap from those very simplified tasks into more adaptive and complex behavioral functions.

Issues of task difficulty and practice remain a major methodologic challenge. We are almost always looking at patients whose performance in any given domain would be worse than the performance of controls, and would also very likely differ in kind as well as in quality. Additionally, that will translate into performance being more effortful and consciously mediated than it will be for controls, which will introduce a number of difficulties in interpretation of data, whether it comes from functional neuroimaging or from other types of investigation.

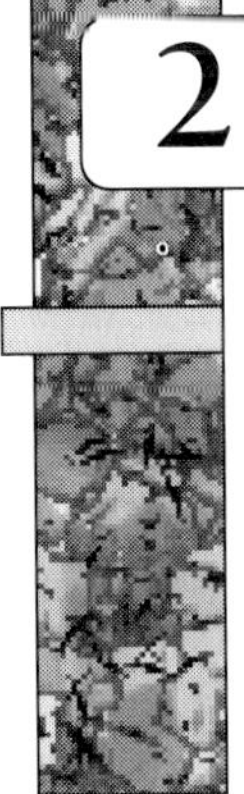

2

Neurorehabilitation Research Opportunities for Improvement and Restoration of Function

Theodore M. Cole, M.D., and James S. Lieberman, M.D.

Medical rehabilitation (physiatry, or physical medicine and rehabilitation) is one of the fastest growing areas in medicine (1). The field was begun before World War II by people from a variety of medical areas in order to provide injured war veterans with better than domiciliary care before their anticipated deaths. But instead of dying as expected, people with conditions such as spinal cord and head injury began to survive, primarily as the result of medical advances such as the development of antibiotics. Their care initially was largely empirical and anecdotal; whatever worked was used to remobilize these individuals.

Medical rehabilitation may be defined as restoring or bringing to a condition of health for useful and constructive activity, usually involving learning new ways to do functions that were lost (2). Broadly speaking, traditional rehabilitation has been an after-the-fact phenomenon: the patient has a pathophysiologic problem that resulted in an impairment, and some kind of intervention is done after that impairment has become fixed. Indeed, much of the discussion in this volume focuses on the patient who has already sustained an insult. However, we are now entering an era in which that definition should probably be changed. Modern interventional techniques applied in the acute phase following a neural injury or insult, either to restore lost function or to *prevent the loss of function,* might well be considered rehabilitation on a continuum that begins with acute intervention.

An example would be some of the acute pharmacologic interventions used to treat stroke patients to restore circulation. This could broaden the concept of rehabilitation to include interventions that begin at the time of insult. Functional neuroimaging, and even traditional neuroimaging, has certainly played a role in this changing approach.

As rehabilitation professionals, we do not think we can do our work, nor serve a patient well, unless we consider the environment in which they live. The field has always concerned itself with the environment in which a patient functions as well as with medical interventions. We must be as concerned with psychological, social, educational, and vocational issues as we are with medical issues; indeed, we consider these issues to be co-equal with medical ones. It is impossible to rehabilitate a patient outside of the context of his or her life.

Neurorehabilitation is an important aspect of the general field of medical rehabilitation—in most in-patient rehabilitation units, one-half to two-thirds of the patients are there because of a neurologic insult. One of the many ideas that abound in rehabilitation intervention is that of restoration of function. In the broad sense, we restore function when we change a patient's ability to interact with his environment. However, this is quite different from restoring function in a patient with a permanent neurologic impairment, such as hemiplegia.

Rehabilitation as a field has been criticized for not having adequate scientific underpinnings beneath its patient assessments, therapies, and interventions. To a large extent the field has remained an anecdotal one, dependent on observing patients going through a rehabilitation process. As a result, when those of us in the field have been asked "what is the science that supports this or that approach?," we have been hard pressed to provide answers.

Biomedical research traditionally has focused on ever-smaller particles of life to yield greater understanding of health and disease. It is important to recognize that the medical rehabilitation research paradigm differs from this traditional approach in many important ways and to recognize that most of the questions faced by the practitioners of medical rehabilitation are not effectively answered by traditional research approaches. Furthermore, problems faced by disabled children and adults are more often related to how their entire body functions within society.

Medical rehabilitation belongs exclusively to no single specialty. Clinicians and scientists contribute to the field from backgrounds as diverse as physiatry, neurology, urology, neurosurgery, orthopedic surgery, internal medicine, physical and occupational therapy, medical engineering, speech and language pathology, and neuropsychology. Progress in the medical sciences has led to a longer life expectancy, higher survival rate from trauma and disease, and an increasing population of Americans with moderate to severe disabilities. Disabilities consume 6.5 percent of the U.S. gross national product, and one out of every seven of us has, or will have, a significant disability. About 4 percent of the U.S. population have disabilities so severe that they are unable to function in a major activity appropriate to their age group, and face major impediments in quality of life (3).

The National Center for Medical Rehabilitation Research has identified several research priorities for funding in the next cycle:

- functional mobility;
- behavioral adaptation to disability, i.e., the response of the whole person to treatment, not just organ responses;
- assistive technology; and
- measurement of treatment effectiveness.

This volume relates directly to several of these research priorities, and it is hoped that it will encourage research that will benefit the disabled person's functional mobility, behavior, and local and general body response to treatment.

The World Health Organization has developed a system called the ICIDH—International Classification of Impairment, Disease, and Handicap (4). In this concept, a *disease* may lead to an *impairment,* which may lead to a *disability,* and this in turn may lead to a *handicap* or disadvantage in life roles. The paradigm accepted by the new National Center for Medical Rehabilitation Research within the National Institute of Child Health and Human Development emphasizes five domains of scientific research: pathophysiology, impairment, functional limitation, disability, and societal handicap (5).

- *Pathophysiology* is the interruption of or interference with normal physiological and developmental processes or structure.
- *Impairment* that results from that pathology is a loss or abnormality of cognitive, emotional, physiologic, or anatomic structure or function; it includes all losses or abnormalities, not just those attributable to the initial pathophysiology.
- *Functional limitation* is a restriction or lack of an ability to perform an action in the manner, or within the range, consistent with the organ or organ system. This level defines losses in human function that result from the pathophysiology and the impairment.
- *Disability* is an inability or limitation in performing tasks, activities, or roles to levels expected in normal social context; this level is concerned with the interface between the person and society.
- *Societal limitation* is defined as restriction attributable to social policy or barriers. Barriers may be structural or attitudinal; they limit fulfillment of role or deny access to services and opportunities that are associated with full participation in society.

To put this concept into perspective, the *pathology* of occlusive vascular disease might lead to the development of a gangrenous leg. A resulting *impairment* would be an amputation that results in *functional limitations* in walking and other activities. A typical *disability* would be the inability to return to a job requiring a great deal of walking. *Societal limitations* might include the inability to access health care or a limitation in an insurance policy that will not cover the necessary prosthesis, resulting in reduced ability to function in society.

Intervention might be directed at the level of the pathology, the impairment, the disability, or the handicap. Patient outcome may also be measured as changes at any of these levels. In a simple one-to-one relationship, intervention at the level of pathology may produce a change in the pathology, with the outcome seen at that same level. It is also possible that intervention at the level of pathology may produce an effect further downstream, e.g., at the level of impairment, disability, or handicap. Unfortunately, it is difficult to know exactly what influence an intervention at the level of pathology has on the higher levels of functional limitation or disability. It is unlikely that an intervention at disability or societal limitation levels will affect the impairment or pathology levels. Interventions at any level tend to affect levels further along the paradigm.

As an example, consider an individual who has multiple but related pathologies; for example, stroke, diabetic neuropathy, deconditioning, and cataracts. After interventions we must observe the spectrum. We need to know whether the person is working, whether his or her living situation provides maximal independence, and whether he or she is able to recreate as desired.

There are multiple levels of concern between an initial pathophysiology and human function. For example, one might need to climb stairs in order to live and recreate. In order to climb stairs, one needs adequate muscle tone, sense of balance, strength, proprioceptive ability, and depth perception, any one of which might be affected by changes in one or more of these multiple pathologies.

In order to make changes in one's handicap, we need to see relationships between pathology and disability. It is hoped that functional imaging of the diseased and injured nervous system will make a substantial contribution to progress in managing these clinical problems by providing a better understanding of disabling conditions and their responses to traditional and emerging treatments. Rehabilitation investigators must communicate the functional problems faced by disabled people to their colleagues in the imaging sciences to better focus neuroimaging research on patients' problems.

At this time, we lack sufficient understanding of the normal parameters of *in vivo* nervous structure and related function, especially as they are influenced by age and gender. We do not know what opportunities may exist to help us improve or restore human function by applying information gained from functional neuroimaging. However, the following are suggested:

1. Functional neuroimaging can help to establish normal anatomic and physiologic parameters.
2. Functional neuroimaging can establish diagnostic indices for the brain, the spinal cord, and peripheral structures, which will help us better understand pathophysiologic processes and thus specific disabilities.
3. Functional neuroimaging may help to predict the viability of diseased parts of the nervous system in order to prudently allocate expensive technologies. Predictions for prognosis can also help the clinician manage ongoing therapies.
4. Functional neuroimaging has the potential to help in the selection of patients for specific treatments. Heretofore we have selected patients based almost entirely on diagnostic category or a defined disability. We may learn that patients should be selected on other bases in order to maximally benefit from a wide range of interventions.
5. Functional neuroimaging has promise for assisting in therapy selection. Whether a therapy is pharmacologic, physical, cognitive, or other, we currently have little insight that allows us to confidently select a beneficial therapy or avoid an unwanted side-effect.
6. Functional neuroimaging can provide measures to assist the clinician in administering therapy. Although we know a considerable amount about dosages of ionizing radiation or toxic drugs, we know much less about other modalities of therapy, including physical interventions, e.g., when they should be initiated, how intensively they should be used, in what order or sequence they should be delivered, or for how long they should be continued.
7. Functional neuroimaging will also help provide a better understanding about drug binding sites upon nervous tissues to provide a better understanding of how and where they work.

8. Functional neuroimaging is a promising tool for monitoring patients undergoing specific treatments by relating changes in structure to clinical response over time. Morphometry, through neuroimaging, is an exciting development that has recently come out of the laboratory and into the clinic.

9. Functional neuroimaging can help us better measure the outcomes of specific treatments. Several technologies offer insights into spontaneous versus therapy-related changes in neural function.

10. Research must relate outcomes to the growing interest in health care-related quality of life, a concept that we are increasingly hearing about as we change our health care systems. We can impact quality of life through better use of science, better selection of patients and therapies, and better monitoring of our results. The long chain of events along the path from diagnosis through treatment to outcome may be better understood using the new tools of functional neuroimaging.

Most of the new procedures now in use in the field have not been subjected to rigorous scientific analysis. As noted by Basmajian (1975), almost all therapeutic procedures used in rehabilitation were anecdotally derived without having been subjected to adequate outcome studies. To some extent that is still true. Rehabilitation providers, consumers, and third party payers do not have answers substantiated by research to such questions as: What are the chances that a given intervention will improve function? What are adverse effects of this treatment, either clinically, physiologically, or structurally? How does one treatment compare with another in terms of efficacy? Shendale (1981) stated that present research in rehabilitation fails to answer some of the most crucial problems with respect to disabled persons and their rehabilitation, and thus falls short of providing adequate answers when rehabilitation professionals must make the kinds of choices that will have to be made in health care in the future.

The research interests of rehabilitation medicine are broad, extending from the molecular level to how people function in their physical and social environment. To professionals in rehabilitation, these are equally important. The NIH Task Force Report on Medical Rehabilitation Research has identified three needs that are critically important to the progress of the field of rehabilitation in the future.

- The field must develop meaningful, quantitative measures of impairments, disabilities, and handicaps, and of the outcomes of our interventions.
- The field must develop standards and guidelines for the design and application of its evaluative tools if we are to achieve consistency and uniformity of effort. We have been hampered by the lack of a common language in rehabilitation medicine, particularly with respect to objective outcomes measures, a deficiency seen throughout all of medicine. Medical rehabilitation has begun to develop such tools and thus is in a good position to further explore measurement sciences as they relate to chronic disease and impairment.
- Finally, we must be able to evaluate the effectiveness of existing and emerging rehabilitation procedures, both at the societal and at the structural and physiologic/biochemical/functional levels. We should focus on how functional neuroimaging can help us to achieve these goals.

The task force listed a number of general priorities, two of which bear on the topic of this volume. One is that of neurophysiologic dysfunction, the broad category of neurologic rehabilitation and neurologic problems. The other is geriatric rehabilitation. A number of problems that are neurophysiologic in nature have generally been considered to be geriatric problems. How might these areas relate to functional neuroimaging?

- We must investigate pharmacologic agents and therapeutic mechanisms that might reduce the extent of neuronal damage or death caused by disease or injury. A description of the sequence of the physiologic and biologic events that can lead to cell death or survival in the nervous system would provide key basic information.
- We need to define the molecular, cellular, and systemic mechanisms that influence neuronal reorganization and other elements of functional plasticity of the nervous system, and then determine whether functional plasticity can be induced by the chronic administration of pharmacologic agents and/or physical interventions.
- We need to define the mechanisms of motor skill acquisition and learning in both the normal nervous system and a nervous system that has been injured.
- We must investigate and define the potential of interventions such as functional electrical stimulation as treatments for sensory and motor impairments.
- We must develop discriminating, quantitative tests for testing the capacity for and the ability to perform voluntary muscular activities. The more functional the neuroimaging test is, the more it is likely to provide useful information.

A number of general basic and clinical research priorities were suggested by the task force for specific neurologic categories, including stroke, traumatic brain injury, spinal cord injury, demyelinating disease, and neuromuscular disease. Many of these priorities bear, directly or indirectly, upon the following conditions.

Spinal Cord Injury

Some examples of clinical priorities that deal with restoration of function in the area of spinal cord injury include:

- identification of pharmacologic agonists and antagonists that can selectively modulate activation and inhibition of the involved motor pools, so that the motor deficits caused by specific neural impairments can be addressed;
- characterization of the short- and long-term effects of physical interventions such as weight supporting, stepping movements, and so on to determine the neurophysiologic and neurochemical mechanisms involved;
- characterization of the short- and long-term effects of sensory and muscle stimulation and biofeedback on motor capacity; and
- investigation of the interactive effects of pharmacologic, locomotor, and stimulation interventions on locomotor capacity.

Geriatrics

Some considerations from the field of geriatrics are directly applicable to this volume, including epidemiologic studies to determine the relationship between aging and the onset of disabling conditions. Is it possible to predict that a person will have a problem based on certain objective parameters? Can we identify factors that influence the progression or regression of functional limitations that commonly occur as part of the normal aging process? Can we identify and define physiologic and environmental risk factors for falls, limited mobility, and diminished control over fine movements? In other words, what happens in the normal aging nervous system in the absence of trauma or disease? We must investigate neuroplasticity in the nervous and muscular systems of older adults to determine whether it differs from that of younger adults or children, and thus determine whether specific interventions might improve function, particularly with respect to cognitive and neuromotor deficits.

The geriatric area is particularly relevant to the study of cognitive deficits and cognitive rehabilitation in a wide range of disorders such as traumatic brain injury. We must identify the factors responsible for the commonly observed differential between the functional capacity of older adults and their actual level of performance. We also need to develop valid, reliable measures of daily function, and to study the influence of social support mechanisms and a number of other social areas that are not specifically related to neuroimaging. For example, basic research on hormonal, neurochemical, and pharmacologic agents that might improve cognitive and physical function is certainly germane to rehabilitation.

Research can simplistically be divided into two types: descriptive and mechanistic. Rehabilitation research needs improvements in both, and neuroimaging can provide information that will help bridge these areas. It may provide information that is primarily descriptive but it also may bear strongly on mechanistic research. The field must develop accurate and predictive criteria that will help us select the appropriate patient for any particular treatment strategy, whatever its nature.

Rehabilitation is approached in a number of ways. We can help patients to function better in their environment by providing assistive devices or people to minister to their needs. We can teach a patient to substitute for the use of an impaired part of the body by using one that is not impaired. Finally, we can work to provide true restoration of function. At the present time, some combination of these strategies is designed and used for a given patient, who may be independent in certain activities yet require assistance in the performance of others. It is critical that we be able to match a patient with an intervention strategy that will maximize his or her rehabilitation potential; in order to do this, we must be able to accurately assess rehabilitation potential. We use this term both in its traditional sense and to include acute interventions, because the use of imaging studies to determine that a given pathology should be treated with a specific pharmacologic agent involves a form of this matching. Patients who are not suitable candidates for that agent based on neuroimaging data may instead be predicted to require a physical type of intervention.

Another area of descriptive research concerns outcome assessment and its correlation with changes in neuroimaging parameters. A typical rehabilitation research controversy that neuroimaging may help to resolve is whether or not speech pathology assists in the restoration of language skills after a patient becomes aphasic. Some believe this intervention to be beneficial, while others believe that natural recovery and normal neuroplasticity are responsible for improvements in function.

Rehabilitation medicine has a large number of neurophysiologic therapeutic methods that are believed to produce developmental, proprioceptive, or neuromuscular facilitation by altering the neurophysiology of motor function. There is some degree of skepticism as to whether these systems work, and there is certainly a degree of skepticism as to whether they are any better than traditional physical therapy that involves range of motion exercises, mobility training, and the training of normal limbs. Neuroimaging can also help to investigate these systems of therapy.

From a mechanistic research standpoint, areas that seem to be especially promising include neuroimaging techniques that can help us to better understand the mechanisms of learning after neural insult (as well as mechanisms of learning before neural insult), the evaluation of neuroplasticity of motor, language, and cognitive function, and the determination of any changes in learning or plasticity that are specific to the aging brain. Neuroimaging techniques can be expected to be valuable in the evaluation of both the efficacy and the mechanisms of physical and pharmacologic interventions.

Traditional rehabilitation, particularly inpatient rehabilitation as we practice it at this time, is time-intensive, labor-intensive, and expensive. It involves relatively long lengths of stay and the administration of three to five hours of therapy a day. We must be able to document accurate predictive assessment of our patients, followed by efficacious treatment parameters that result in an acceptable outcome in a cost-effective manner. If we do not, we will in the future have significant problems in justifying what we want to do for our patients. Modern neuroimaging techniques have the potential to assist us in accomplishing this goal.

References

1. Cole TM. Rehabilitation medicine: a framework for pulmonary rehabilitation. In: *Pulmonary rehabilitation*. New York: Marcel Dekker, in press.
2. DeLisa JA, Martin GM, Currie DM. Rehabilitation medicine: past present, and future. In: DeLisa JA (ed.). *Rehabilitation medicine: principles and practice*. Philadelphia: J.B. Lippincott, 1988:3.
3. Cole TM, Edgerton VR. *Report of the task force on medical rehabilitation research*. Hunt Valley, MD: National Institutes of Health, 1990.
4. World Health Organization. *International classification of impairments, disabilities and handicaps: a manual for classification relating to the consequences of disease*. Geneva: World Health Organization, 1980.
5. *Research plan for the national center for medical rehabilitation research*. U.S. Department of Health and Human Services, Public Health Service, National Institutes of Health. Publication No. 93-3509, March 1993.

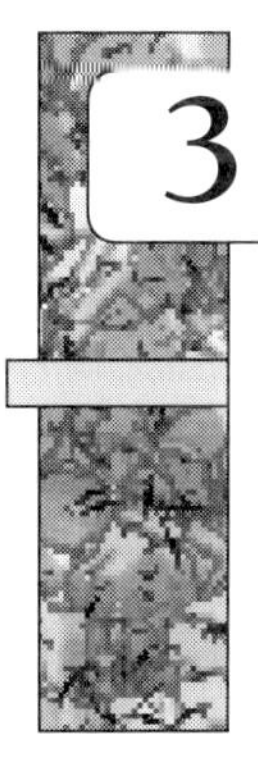

Techniques and Capabilities in SPECT

John W. Keyes, Jr., M.D.

This section introduces the various imaging techniques used for functional imaging of the central nervous system. Although I focus on SPECT (single photon emission computed tomography), I also introduce some of the general topics that are discussed in more detail in some of the other chapters. Let us start by focusing on the word *emission*. Both SPECT and PET (positron emission tomography) are nuclear medicine techniques; that is, they rely on the administration of some sort of radio-labeled material in order to produce the images that we ultimately observe. These images are produced by using special instruments to detect the *emitted* radiation, and this is characteristic of all nuclear medicine procedures. By its very nature, nuclear medicine techniques are functional imaging techniques. They do not measure function in the sense used in neurorehabilitation, but rather in physiologic and metabolic terms. This comes about because a tracer must be chemically tailored to respond to a physiologic process that is localized in a specific area of the body in order to cause the tracer to localize in that area. Although the images produced may look like structural images, there is a functional message that can be extracted from them. That is the essence of functional imaging techniques.

Tomography is a general term used in medical imaging for any technique that produces a cross-sectional image of the body. In SPECT, PET, CT (CAT scanning or computed tomography), and to some extent MRI (magnetic resonance imaging), we produce a cross-sectional image that is almost always transaxial; i.e., at right angles to the long axis (vertical axis) of the body. All of these techniques utilize computer processing of the data that is acquired by the scanning equipment in order to produce and display the final images that are produced. Hence, putting all of these terms together, we have *emission transaxial computed tomography*.

Single photon is a rather poorly chosen term that separates SPECT from PET imaging. It means only that the techniques do not use positron emitting nuclides and the scanning is based on different detection technology than is used for positron imaging. All of these imaging techniques share in common the fact that data is acquired by either moving a detector around the patient or actually surrounding the patient with detector material and acquiring a series of images looking at the patient from a number of different angles around the central axis of the body. The common type of SPECT instruments in use today have an Anger type gamma camera, which rotates around the body while a patient lies on a cantilevered table. In a PET machine, it is more common for the patient to be entirely surrounded by stationary detectors, but in either case the images are produced by detecting the emitted radiation from the patient. In an x-ray CT scanner, there is an x-ray source on one side of the patient and an array of detectors on the other, and these rotate together around the patient, generating x-ray type images of anatomic structure.

SPECT has a number of significant advantages. Primary among these is that it uses conventional radionuclides that are universally available, and it can be performed almost anywhere. Furthermore, all manufacturers of nuclear medicine equipment now produce SPECT scanners.

Another critical point in all of these techniques is that they all rely on a computer system of some sort to take the data produced by the image acquisition end of the system and convert it into the tomographic images that we look at. Because all of this takes place inside a computer, these images are inherently digital; e.g., they are already in numerical form stored inside the computer. The pictures we see are actually an electronic transformation of these digital numbers onto a computer display screen. This is true of most of the imaging techniques that are discussed here.

All manufacturers now produce SPECT instruments. Many of the systems available for nuclear medicine SPECT imaging have been specifically tailored to optimize their performance for SPECT. Often these instruments incorporate two or three detectors rather than one. This approach of using multiple detectors to surround the patient with the imaging apparatus increases sensitivity and also tends to improve the overall image quality. These specialized SPECT machines are currently commercially available and virtually every nuclear medicine laboratory in the United States can provide SPECT imaging.

It is important to realize that all of these modern computed tomographic techniques are inherently three-dimensional imaging techniques. What comes out of a SPECT machine is a series of tomographic slices such as those shown in Figure 3-1. They encompass the entire brain as a series of single slices, starting at the top and working downward through the level of the cerebellum. Although they are produced as a series of two-dimensional transaxial tomographic slices, what is stored in the computer's memory is essentially a three-dimensional image. SPECT, PET, CT, and MRI data all consist of three-dimensional data sets that can be manipulated and interacted with as three-dimensional maps. Figure 3-2 shows one way of dissecting these three-dimensional images from the original transaxial slices into alternative tomographic slices in other orientations. This technique is widely used and allows the viewer to

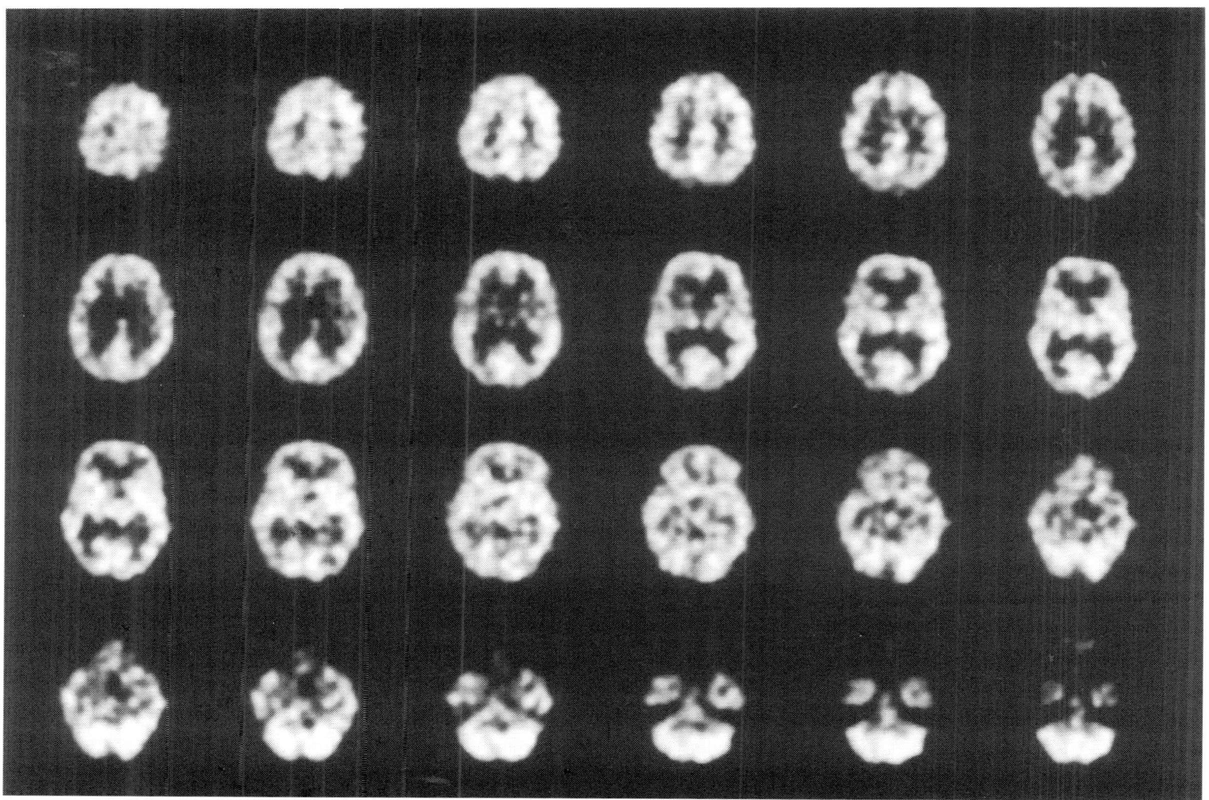

Figure 3-1. Normal HMPAO SPECT brain scan. Images represent contiguous transaxial sections beginning at the vertex (*upper left*) and extending through the cerebellum (*lower right*).

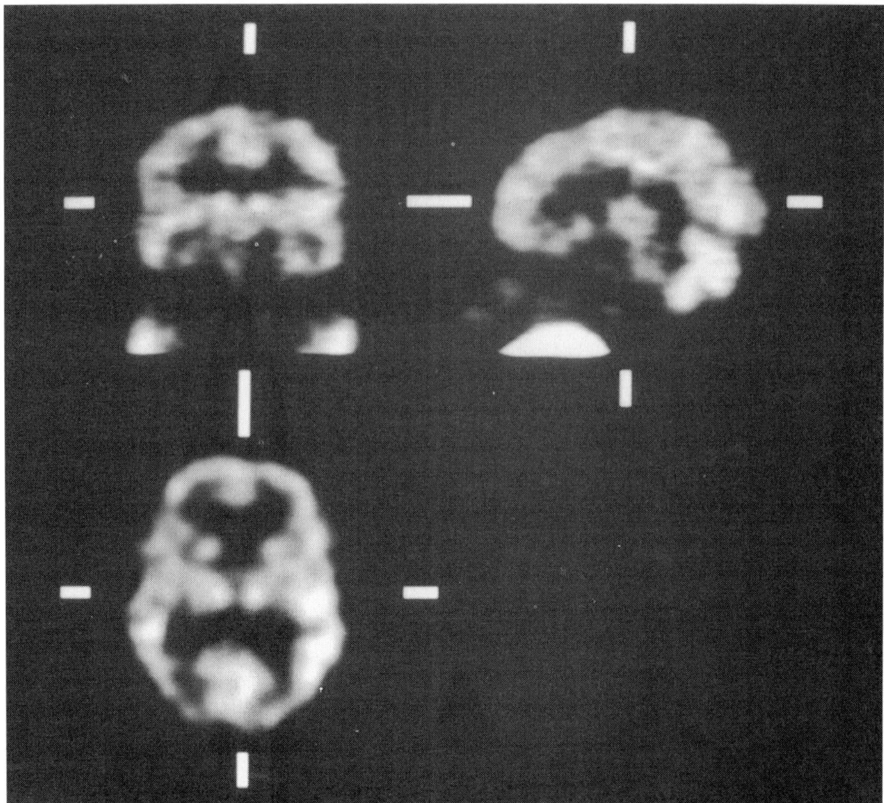

Figure 3-2. The same normal study shown in Figure 3-1, redisplayed to show orthogonal tomographic sections in the coronal and sagittal planes as well as the transaxial plane.

see not only the transaxial slices but also the corresponding coronal or sagittal slices through the brain (Figure 3-3).

There are also other ways of presenting three-dimensional data. Figure 3-4 shows a normal brain scan processed to look truly three-dimensional. There are also some sophisticated computer techniques that permit these three-dimensional images to be played back as movies and for generating what we call reprojection images, which permit the user to view the organ in three dimensions. All of these methods are very useful and provide extremely powerful tools for analyzing these images when we sit down and try to extract meaning from them.

Nuclear Medicine Tracers for SPECT Imaging

What gave the field of nuclear medicine its primary impetus in the early 1960s was brain scanning using tracers that were nothing more than markers for dis-

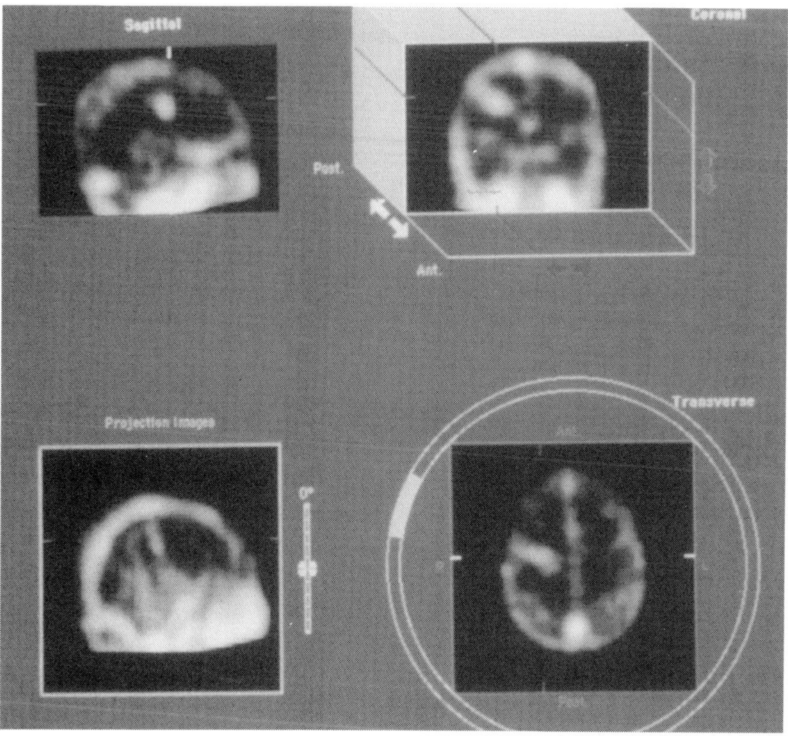

Figure 3-3. The value of using views in multiple orthogonal planes is shown in this study of a patient with a venous angioma. Both the location of the lesion and the large draining vein extending to the meningeal surface of the brain can be seen.

ruption of the blood brain barrier. Although such tracers are not widely used today, having been largely replaced by more advanced structural imaging techniques such as CT and MRI, they do lend themselves quite readily to SPECT techniques and are occasionally useful. Figure 3-5A shows an MRI image of a patient who has an obvious abnormality, which had been thought to be a stroke but when imaged using a blood brain barrier agent and SPECT proved to be a tumor.

Currently, the most widely used tracer for brain imaging in nuclear medicine is Ceretec® or HMPAO. This tracer allows one to generate maps of blood flow to the brain. Blood flow imaging is a powerful tool for two reasons. First, many of the problems that involve disruption of normal neurologic function are related to primary cerebral vascular disease. Obviously, a tracer that looks at brain blood flow is a very direct way of examining any problem associated with its disruption. Of perhaps still greater importance is the tight coupling of brain blood flow to brain function and metabolism. These blood flow imaging agents thus provide a tool to examine brain function at a much more fundamental level than is superficially apparent. This is a kind of "second order" look because a change in function is

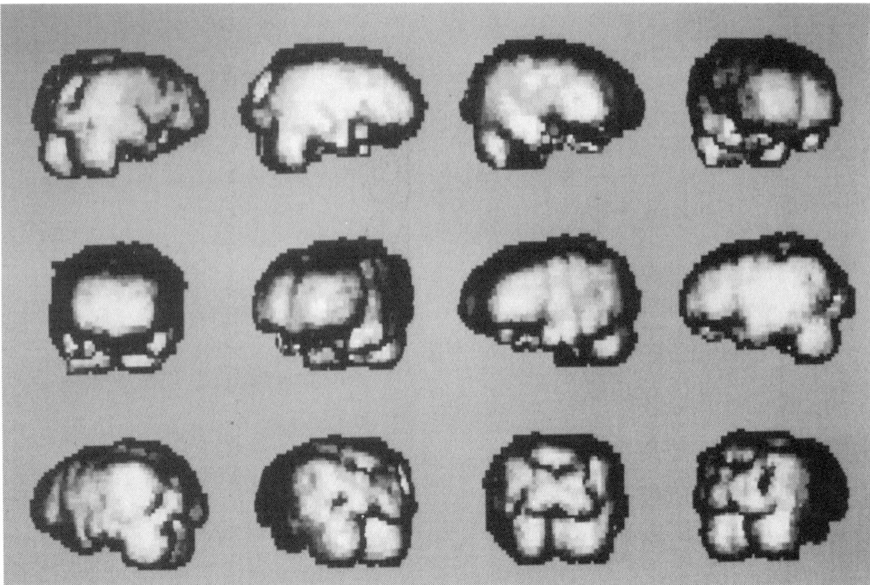

Figure 3-4. Alternative three-dimensional display of a normal HMPAO brain study. In actual practice, each image would be one frame of a movie loop and when displayed on the computer screen the "solid" image would appear to rotate, strongly enhancing the illusion of three-dimensionality.

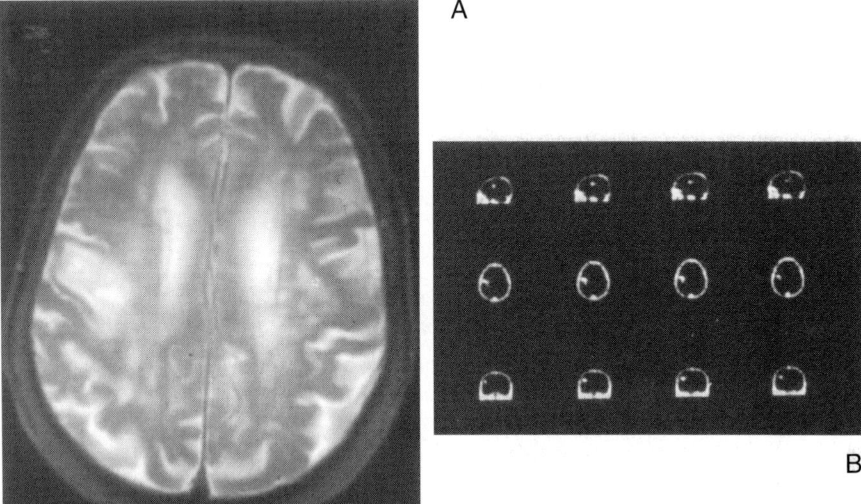

Figure 3-5. (A) MRI of a patient with a distinct right hemisphere lesion thought to be a stroke. (B) SPECT study done with Tc-99m DTPA several months after onset of symptoms. A stroke would not show an abnormality so late after the acute event. This proved to be a glioblastoma.

reflected in a change in metabolic activity, which is then reflected as a change in blood flow. This coupling of blood flow and metabolism allows one to do things with blood flow agents that might not appear immediately possible. Figure 3-6 shows an example of a patient who has had a small stroke involving one of the branches of the left middle cerebral artery. This is an example of using the brain blood flow agent HMPAO to map a problem specifically related to primary cerebral vascular disease. On the other hand, Figure 3-7 shows a patient with senile dementia of the Alzheimer's type. This produces a very characteristic pattern on SPECT imaging (which can also be seen by PET) because of the functional disruption caused by the disease. Images of this sort should not be looked at as structural images, but as functional images that provide a graphic display of the anatomic distribution of functional change.

One of the more widespread uses of SPECT and PET today is in the evaluation of patients who have partial complex epilepsy. Figure 3-8 is an example of studies obtained on a patient with temporal lobe epilepsy using a brain flow agent and SPECT. The dramatic change that occurs from the interictal state to the ictal state is readily apparent on these images.

Images of this sort should be compared with the PET functional images discussed in the next section. It will then be possible to see how these "second order" maps of function compare to direct functional maps of glucose utilization and hence brain function.

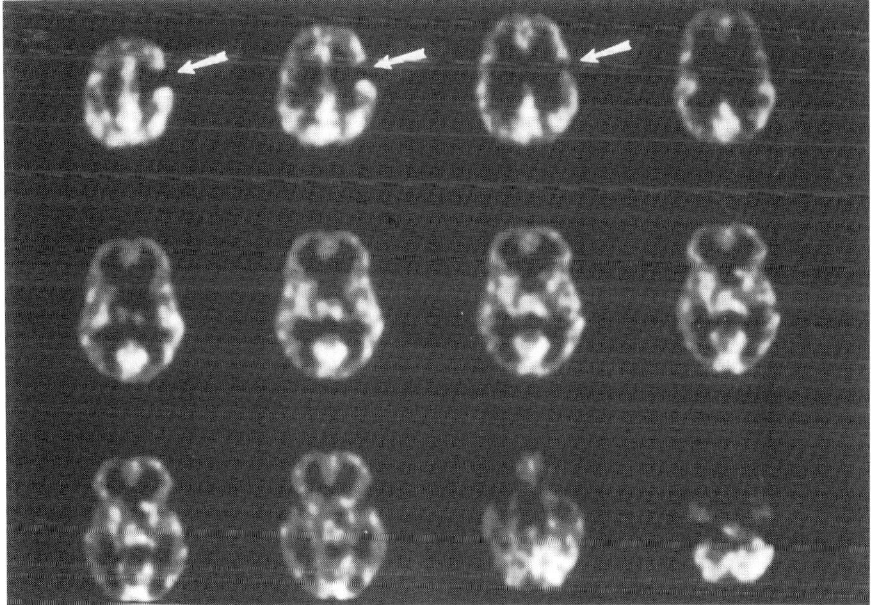

Figure 3-6. HMPAO study of a patient with a small left cerebral stroke *(arrows).*

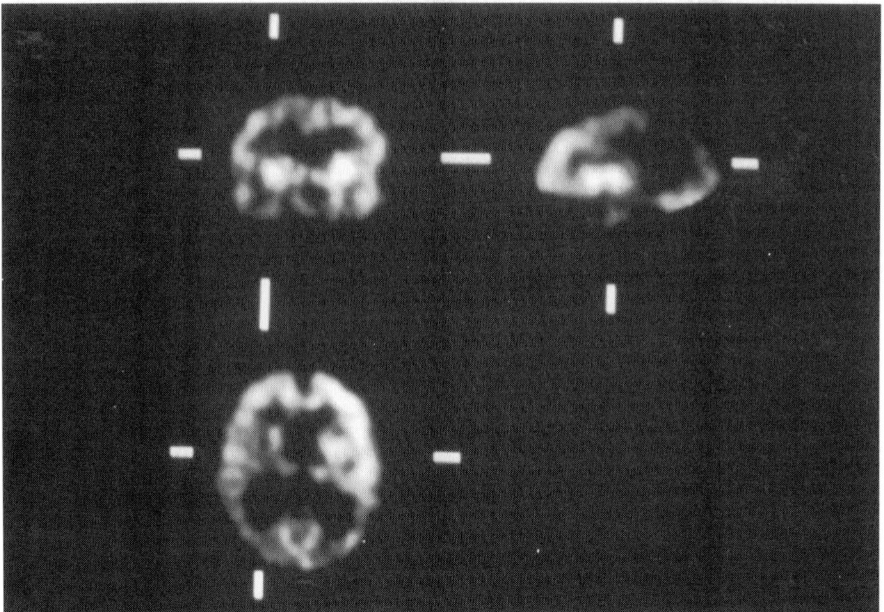

Figure 3-7. HMPAO study in a patient with advanced dementia of the Alzheimer's type. The pronounced decrease in blood flow to the parietal and occipital lobes can be seen. Compare this study with the normal study shown in Figure 3-2.

Other areas can be looked at using SPECT and different tracers. For example, blood volume imaging can be accomplished with a tracer that labels red blood cells. Blood volume imaging is important because one can use multiple tracers as a combination type test in order to extract useful functional information. For example, it has been shown in primary cerebral vascular disease that the relationship of local brain blood volume as imaged with labeled red blood cells compared with local cerebral blood flow imaged with HMPAO provides a much more powerful set of analytic tools for looking at whether there is a completed stroke or simply ischemia and in attempting to determine prognostic outcomes.

A wide range of other tracers are also available. A number of nuclear medicine tracers are specific for neoplasms, although they are not specific for particular tumor types. For example, thallium-201, a tracer that is normally used for evaluating blood flow to the myocardium, is also a rather specific imaging agent for neoplasms in the brain. Why this is true is unclear since it is not a blood–brain barrier agent but is actually specific for neoplasm. Figure 3-9 is an example of this. Figure 3-9A shows a CT study with a large lesion within the brain of a patient with AIDS. The differential diagnostic possibilities include lymphoma and toxoplasmosis. Lesions of both types would be positive using a blood–brain barrier agent

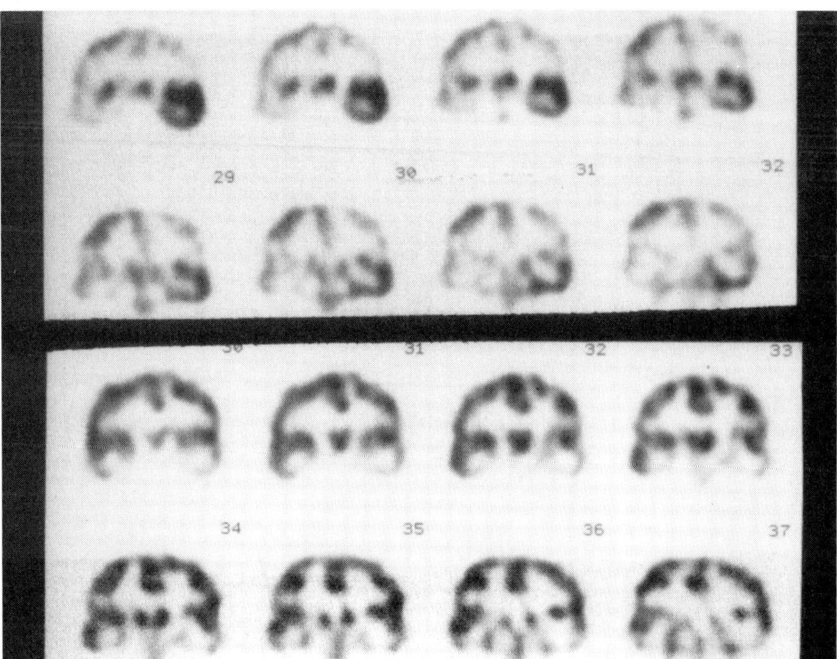

Figure 3-8. (A) Ictal SPECT study (coronal sections) obtained in a patient with left temporal lobe epilepsy. (B) Comparable study obtained during an interictal period. Note the profound change in blood flow to the left temporal lobe that occurs with the seizure.

but thallium uptake is specific for lymphoma, which was present in this patient and is shown in Figure 3-9B.

SPECT agents for imaging a variety of neuroreceptors are under investigation at the present time. Figure 3-10 shows a series of images taken with a D2 dopamine agent labeled with iodine-123. A strong localization of this tracer within the basal ganglia of a normal individual can be readily appreciated.

I have already mentioned the use of multiple tracers in combination. These studies also lend themselves extremely well to use in combination with other imaging techniques. Again, Figure 3-9 is an example of this in which one of the structural imaging techniques has identified an abnormality but the nuclear medicine technique has provided a specific diagnosis.

Conclusion

It can be seen that many of the "high tech" imaging techniques used to visualize the structure and function of the brain share many common features and characteristics. Modern imaging technology permits evaluation of the brain from many

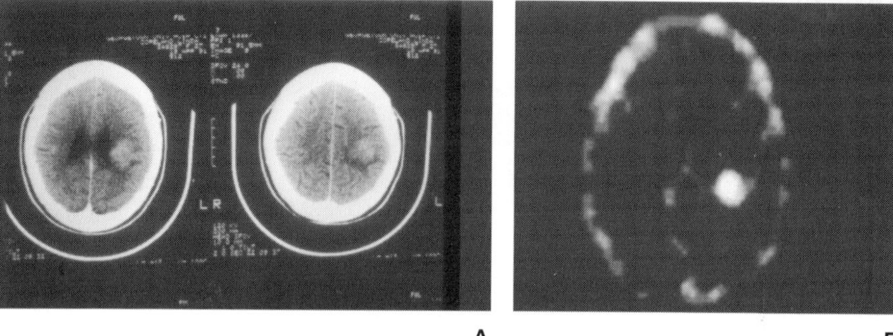

A   B

Figure 3-9. (A) CT images in a patient with AIDS and mental symptoms. The distinct left-sided lesion could represent either lymphoma or toxoplasmosis. (B) T1-201 SPECT study shows intense uptake of tracer in the lesion indicating lymphoma.

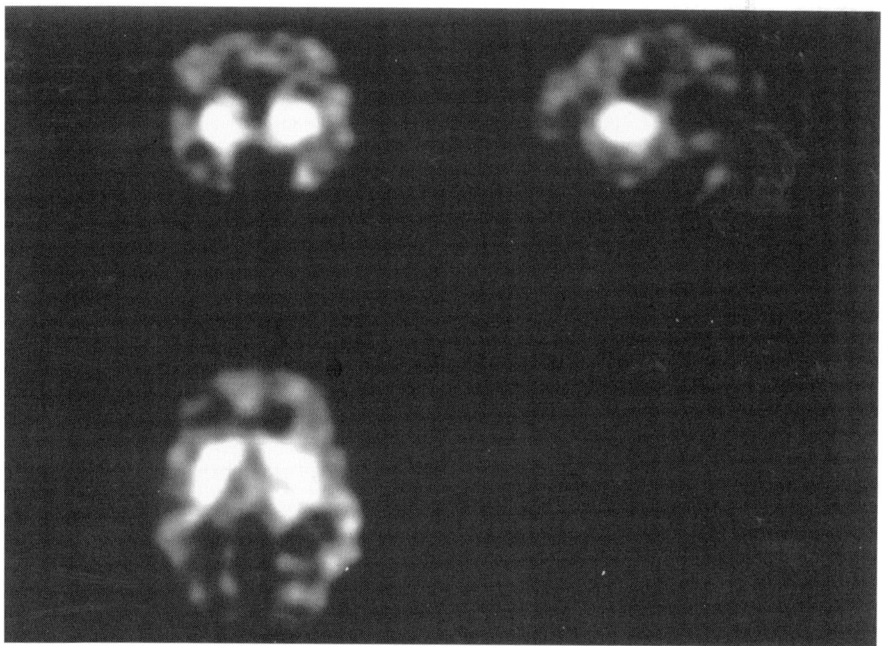

Figure 3-10. SPECT images of an I-123 labeled tracer for D2 dopamine receptors. Note the strong localization within the basal ganglia.

viewpoints and allows this data to be correlated and analyzed in a number of ways. It is a powerful tool to analyze the changes that occur in the brain following an injury or other insult and provides a means to investigate the effects of rehabilitation on brain function.

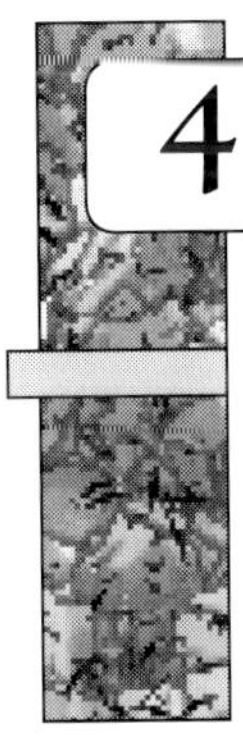

4

Techniques and Capabilities in PET

Sid Gilman, M.D.

Positron emission tomography (PET) provides a means of functional imaging that allows visualization and measurement of a number of chemical processes in the central nervous system. These include cerebral metabolic rates for glucose; cerebral metabolic rates for oxygen; cerebral blood volume; cerebral blood flow; and the density of neurotransmitters and neurotransmitter receptors. The technique is highly flexible and has essentially unlimited capability as new ligands are being developed constantly.

The utility of PET has only begun to be explored in neurologic diseases and has tremendous potential for neurorehabilitation. PET offers the advantage that it can measure functional processes in contrast to structural imaging studies such as CT and MR scanning, which principally allow examination of the anatomy of the brain. Recent developments in MR scanning have made it possible to visualize blood flow both within blood vessels and within brain tissue, and this technique may prove to be helpful in place of or as an adjunct to PET imaging. SPECT (single photon emission computed tomography) is another functional imaging technique that is discussed in Chapter 3. It is less expensive than PET but has the disadvantage of low count numbers because of the need for collimation and difficulty in carrying out quantitative measurements. Nevertheless, the utility of SPECT for rehabilitation is likely to increase with time.

In this chapter, I discuss the capabilities of PET in a variety of neurologic disorders, including dementia, brain tumors, epilepsy, stroke, movement disorders, and ataxias.

A good deal of our information on functional imaging with PET has come from the use of [^{18}F]fluorodeoxyglucose with PET, which provides quantitative measurements of cerebral glucose metabolic rates. This has been used extensively in the dementias. Alzheimer's disease, a progressive neurodegenerative disease of undetermined etiology, causes middle life or late life onset of a slowly progressive dementia. PET studies with fluorodeoxyglucose demonstrate hypometabolism within the posterior parietal and temporal regions early in the disease. PET allows a diagnosis to be made with a high degree of reliability, since the pattern of posterior hemisphere hypometabolism appears to be quite specific for Alzheimer's disease.

Progressive supranuclear palsy (PSP) is another neurodegenerative disorder of undetermined cause presenting with Parkinsonian features but with supranuclear disorders of gaze, cervical rigidity, bradykinesia, and a mild dementia. PET studies of PSP reveal frontal hypometabolism along with decreased metabolic rates in the basal ganglia.

In patients with Parkinson's disease, cerebral glucose metabolic rates are generally within normal limits. Recent studies suggest there may be hypermetabolism in certain structures of the basal ganglia. In patients with Parkinson's disease who become demented, however, PET studies with fluorodeoxyglucose show a pattern that is very similar to that seen in Alzheimer's disease.

Normal pressure hydrocephalus (NPH) is a progressive neurologic disorder characterized by a gait disturbance, urinary incontinence, and dementia resulting from malabsorption of cerebrospinal fluid. PET studies show a diffuse decrease of glucose metabolism through the cerebral hemispheres. One case has been reported in which a pattern analogous to that seen in Alzheimer's disease was found in a patient with NPH. This pattern was reversed after shunting relieved the symptoms.

Multiple infarct dementia (MID) patients show spotty hypometabolism distributed through the cerebral cortex bilaterally in a pattern that is different from that seen in Alzheimer's disease.

Cerebral gliomas usually show glucose hypermetabolism within the tumor, and the distribution effectively outlines the full extent of the tumor. PET studies of glucose metabolism have been augmented by new ligands that are specific for certain kinds of brain tumors. For example, PK 11195 has been used to identify cerebral tumors and appears to be highly specific for gliomas and other disorders in which large amounts of glial tissue are concentrated within the central nervous system. PET with glucose metabolism has proved to be highly effective in differentiating recurrent cerebral tumors from radiation-induced necrosis, which is a frequent clinical disturbance. Typically, a patient treated for a brain tumor some years earlier develops a progressive neurologic disorder. Anatomical imaging studies commonly are not diagnostic. PET studies with fluorodeoxyglucose in this situation demonstrate absence of metabolic activity in patients with postradiation necrosis and hypermetabolism in the area of brain tumor if recurrent tumor is responsible for the new symptoms.

PET studies with fluorodeoxyglucose have been very helpful in the diagnosis of epilepsy and particularly in prescreening patients for surgical treatment of complex partial epilepsy. Patients with this disorder show focal hypometabolism interictally within the area responsible for the ictal events. Many patients have multiple areas of hypometabolism, and these patients are not good candidates for ablative surgery. When a single hypometabolic zone is found in the temporal lobe, the chances that a patient will benefit by surgery are enhanced. Studies of cerebral blood flow have successfully captured epileptic events and shown marked increases of blood flow within the regions that are hypometabolic during the interictal period.

PET studies of cerebral blood flow and blood volume have demonstrated that severe carotid stenosis or occlusion results in reactive vasodilation in the ipsilateral cerebral hemisphere. PET studies of cerebral blood flow, cerebral metabolic rate for oxygen, and cerebral metabolic rate for glucose within forty-eight hours of cerebral infarction in most patients have showm reduced cerebral blood flow, raised oxygen extraction, reduced metabolic rate for oxygen, and reduced metabolic rate for glucose. Some patients show normal blood flow, reduced oxygen extraction rate, reduced oxygen metabolic rate, and normal glucose metabolic rate. With completed cerebral infarction, PET studies show decreases in blood flow, oxygen, and glucose metabolism in a much larger volume of tissue than with anatomical imaging studies. PET studies also reveal remote effects from diaschisis. Following infarction in the precentral area of the cerebral cortex, a decrease in glucose metabolism occurs in the contralateral cerebellar hemisphere even though the cerebellum is not structurally affected.

In summary, PET helps determine whether infarction has occurred in patients with transient ischemic attacks and the size of infarction in patients presumed to have fully recovered from stroke. PET provides a valuable means of following stroke in evolution. It reveals the full extent of tissue injury, including remote effects, when anatomical imaging studies show only local changes. Clinical symptoms tend to correlate more closely with PET than with CT or MR results. PET studies in the future will be important in evaluating new therapies in stroke. Examples of this include TPA, glutamate antagonists, and the effects of various surgical procedures, including carotid endarterectomy.

I turn now to discuss the utility of PET in movement disorders. Huntington's disease is a progressive neurodegenerative disease inherited as an autosomal dominant trait. The responsible gene has now been identified and cloned. The disease begins in middle age, after the child-bearing years. Both sexes are affected, and the major neuropathological changes are in the striatum. Clinical symptoms consist of choreic movements with progressive dementia and severe depression. PET studies with glucose show primarily hypometabolism in the caudate nucleus and putamen. About one-third of presymptomatic subjects have hypometabolism, and there is a close match between genetic studies and PET studies in the at-risk subjects who have been examined so far. PET studies show normal uptake of fluorodopa in striatal presynaptic dopaminergic terminals and decreased density of D2 receptors as studied with PET and methylspiperone. I urge caution about interpretation of these studies since the models for these ligands are not very good.

Wilson's disease is a progressive systemic and neurologic disorder inherited as an autosomal recessive trait. The onset is in childhood, adolescence, or adulthood, and both sexes are affected. The clinical symptoms result principally from deposition of copper in liver and brain, and in brain the lenticular nuclei are particularly affected. Kayser-Fleischer rings can be seen in the corneas of symptomatic patients. PET studies show diffusely reduced glucose metabolism in the frontal and parietal cortex, the frontal and parietal white matter, the basal ganglia, and the cerebellar hemispheres.

Next, I will touch on PET studies in the ataxias. PET studies with fluorodeoxyglucose of paraneoplastic cerebellar degeneration show widespread hypometabolism throughout the central nervous system. Patients with alcoholic cerebellar degeneration show reduced glucose metabolism in the anterior superior vermis of the cerebellum. Olivopontocerebellar atrophy is one of the most common adult-onset ataxias. It is a progressive degenerative disease that occurs sporadically and in an inherited form with dominant or recessive transmission. Involvement of both sexes is common, and usually the onset is in middle age. The disease is characterized clinically by a gradually progressive ataxia of gait, an ataxic dysarthria, incoordination of the limbs, and nystagmus. Dementia occurs only in some hereditary cases of OPCA. The neuropathology consists of degeneration of neurons with reactive gliosis in the inferior olives, pons, and cerebellum. Glial and neuronal cytoplasmic inclusions have been described in sporadic cases. PET studies show a generalized decrease of metabolic rate, although it is maximal in the brain stem and cerebellum, with decreased blood flow in the same sites. Studies of GABA-A/benzodiazepine receptors with [11C]flumazenil and PET show decreased influx of ligand (K_1), but only slightly decreased receptor distribution volume in the cerebellum, basal ganglia, and cerebral cortex. This finding suggests that pharmacological intervention utilizing these preserved receptors may ameliorate the symptoms of this disease.

Multiple system atrophy is a disorder related to sporadic OPCA. MSA is an adult-onset progressive degenerative disease of undetermined cause affecting both sexes. The term MSA currently includes striatonigral degeneration, Shy-Drager syndrome, and some cases of sporadic OPCA. These patients present with extrapyramidal symptoms that are levodopa unresponsive or poorly responsive, autonomic insufficiency, or cerebellar signs. The manner of onset is highly variable. Some present initially with extrapyramidal symptoms, others with cerebellar disorders, and some with autonomic insufficiency. The neuropathology in these patients includes degeneration of neurons and reactive gliosis in the striatum, inferior olives, brainstem, cerebellum, and intermediolateral columns of the spinal cord. Glial and neuronal cytoplasmic argentophilic inclusions are found throughout the brain. PET studies with fluorodeoxyglucose show decreased cerebral metabolic rate in the cerebral cortex, basal ganglia, thalamus, cerebellum, and brainstem. PET studies with [18F]fluorodopa show decreased uptake in the striatum. PET studies with [11C]raclopride show decreased binding to D2 receptors in the striatum. We have found in PET studies with [11C]flumazenil that GABA-A/benzodiazepine receptors are preserved in MSA. This indicates that some of the symptoms of MSA might be ameliorated with medications targeted to these receptors.

Friedreich's ataxia is a progressive degenerative disease inherited as an autosomal recessive trait with onset in childhood or adolescence. Early in the disease these patients show widespread glucose hypermetabolism, and as the disease progresses, cerebral glucose metabolic rates return toward normal.

Finally, I would like to show some exciting preliminary data obtained with [11C]raclopride, a substance that can be used with PET to measure striatal D2 binding. We have studied only a limited number of patients, and the results obviously are preliminary. We found decreased binding in multiple system atrophy, normal binding in sporadic olivopontocerebellar atrophy, and decreased binding in supranuclear palsy. A substantial number of people with Alzheimer's disease develop extrapyramidal symptoms, the pathogenesis of which is uncertain. The possibilities include degeneration of nigrostriatal fibers, striatal neurons, or other sites. We studied raclopride binding in patients with Alzheimer's disease, who show normal levels of binding. In contrast, in Alzheimer's disease with extrapyramidal symptoms, a marked decrease of binding is found. This suggests that there is a decrease of striatal D2 receptor density, and this may be relevant to the pathogenesis of extrapyramidal symptoms in Alzheimer's disease.

I will summarize briefly by pointing out that first, we have limited means to evaluate brain function, and second, that many techniques of determining brain physiology and pathology are indirect. The neurological history and examination, CSF, and EEG are all indirect techniques. Anatomical imaging studies give information primarily about brain structure but not function. Direct visualization of brain tissue at surgery involves the risk of cerebral injury. In contrast, PET provides direct information about cerebral blood flow, blood volume, cerebral metabolic rate for glucose and oxygen, and the density of specific neurotransmitter terminals and receptors. In many clinical situations, PET provides highly important and, at times, cost-effective information for the evaluation of dementia, epilepsy, and brain tumors.

5

The Potential of Magnetic Source Imaging (MSI) in Neurorehabilitation

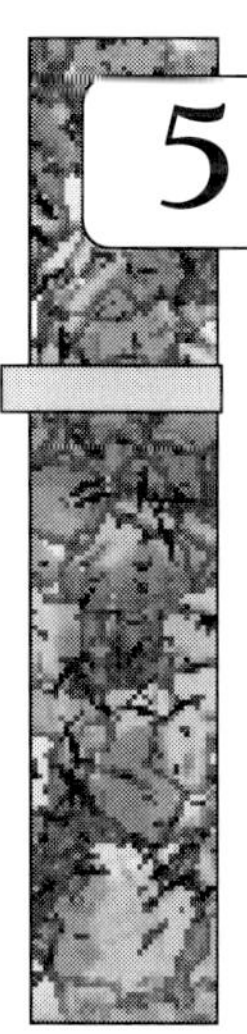

Barry J. Schwartz, Ph.D., Tony T. Yang, M.D., Ph.D.,
Christopher C. Gallen, M.D., Ph.D., and
Floyd E. Bloom, M.D.

Introduction: Functional Imaging and Neurorehabilitation

An obvious goal of applying functional imaging to the measurement of neurorehabilitation is to localize the neural processing substrate that underlies the brain's response to injury, especially to track its still mysterious capacity for recovery of function. The ideal would be to obtain a physiological prognosis for the progress of rehabilitation. For example, functional imaging technology would monitor recovery in a patch of cortex rendered temporarily dysfunctional, as in the case of a transient ischemic attack or head trauma. It would detect a change in location of function that may be in the process of "migrating," as it were, from an injured area to another area previously not associated with it, a process that may prove to mediate the recovery of motor control after massive stroke. Rapid advancements have occurred in the arsenal of tools being readied to accomplish these seemingly utopian tasks, comprising early but real steps toward building a set of practical tools for guiding the neurorehabilitator of the future. Magnetic source imaging (MSI) is a means of measuring neural activity directly and noninvasively. Preliminary clinical results using MSI suggest a role for this technology alongside functional MR and PET/SPECT methods.

Magnetoencephalography and Magnetic Source Imaging

Magnetic source imaging is a product of combining magnetoencephalographic (MEG) measurement and source localization with MR or CT images, using a common frame of reference. MSI is a rapid and noninvasive method of drawing a spatial map of the neural sources of spontaneous events and rhythms, or of evoked sensory and cognitive measurements. MSI maps may include information about sensory and motor function.

as well as maps indicating known signals of dysfunction, such as interictal spikes in epilepsy or focal slowing associated with cortical injury (1).

The human cerebral magnetic field is exceedingly small, on the order of 50–250 femtoTesla (fT, 10^{-15} Tesla), and recordings of this field must occur in the context of substantial noise including the earth 70×10^9 fT, the surrounding laboratory and urban environment (10^{14} fT), and nearby MRI scanners (1.5×10^{15} fT). The small signal and huge noise currently require very sensitive superconducting quantum interference device based detectors (SQUID) and a magnetically shielded room. MEG works by detecting tiny magnetic field changes that are caused by intracellular currents, in particular the rapidly fluctuating, graded changes of post-synaptic potentials (PSPs). The spatial summation of PSPs within the long, closely packed palisades of cortical pyramidal cells results in net currents producing magnetic fields detectable at the surface of the scalp with sensitive instruments. These neuromagnetic fields pass through brain, cerebrospinal fluid, skull, and scalp relatively undistorted and unattenuated due to the fact that their magnetic permeability, unlike their electrical conductivity, is nearly the same at unity. By comparison, the spatial pattern of electrical potentials measured by EEG on the scalp have been subject to the distorting influence of the 80:1 ratio of impedances of skull to brain and CSF, and by the preferential flow of electrons toward sutures and openings in the skull. An EEG electrode pair placed at any location may pick up the fields emanating from sources throughout the brain, a factor that greatly limits the spatial selectivity of the measurements. The spatial precision of MEG is such that 1 mm size artificial electrical sources placed inside realistic head-shaped mechanical models measured and overlaid on MR scans, were shown to be accurate to within 1–2 millimeters (2).

With signal averaging, MEG evoked fields from repeated sensory stimulation can be summed and detected outside the head. Most MSI studies to date have used the single equivalent current dipole (ECD) model for source localization. This model is best suited to situations in which the brain signal is dominated by activity from a single source, as might occur during the peak of an epileptic spike or an evoked potential. At selected times in relation to the stimulus, these fields can be adequately modeled as compact ECD sources, reflecting the intracellular current flow associated with specific sensory events. Since the magnetic field is perpendicular to the direction of current flow, MEG tends to be most sensitive to sources oriented tangentially to the skull surface, as, for example, in the folds of cortical sulci. MEG is also selective to neocortex because it is insensitive to radial current sources, including current sources emanating from central, subcortical structures (3).

Unlike electroencephalography (EEG), MSI is reference-free. Although MSI results are spatially precise relative to EEG, PET, SPECT, and fMRI, MSI is highly selective to cortex and to sources tangential to the skull, which is to say that MEG is insensitive to radial and central signals. MSI is thus strongly complementary to other imaging techniques. While the temporal precision of MSI is as fine as EEG, MSI can also localize separate neural events occurring two to three orders of magnitude faster than changes in blood oxygenation or regional metabolism. The combination represents a technology that can monitor millisecond by millisecond alterations in the activity in regions of cortex separated by as little as a few millimeters, regions as compact as one square millimeter, and containing as few as 20,000 to 50,000 simultaneously active neurons summating post-synaptic potentials (4,5). MSI thus opens up the possibility of localizing and tracking temporal sequences of activity in functional neural subunits, sequences tied to distinctive physiological processing operations that may be altered by injury, and which may alter in characteristic ways in the process of recovering functionality.

Clinical Applications of MSI Measurements

MSI has been employed to detect abnormal or pathological spontaneous events, including focal slowing associated with mass lesions (6,7) and interictal spikes associated with epilepsy, in order to aid in the planning of surgery for patients with seizures uncontrolled by drugs (8–10). Additionally, MSI has provided precise, noninvasive maps of functional areas of somatosensory and motor cortex for use by neurosurgeons to localize eloquent cortex in cases subject to distortion due to mass effects of tumors or edema prior to surgery (11–13).

The neuromagnetic measurements described below were conducted on a Magnes® Biomagnetometer (Biomagnetic Technologies, Inc.), with thirty-seven detector channels arrayed in a series of three concentric circles around a central detector (Figure 5-1). The array diameter is 144 mm. Intrinsic noise in each channel is <10fT/Hz. The probe is typically placed over a location assessed as relevant to the signal of interest and may be moved after initial recordings to the most optimal location. MEG functional localizations were calculated in a three-dimensional coordinate system based on standard extracranial fiducial markers (left and right preauricular points and nasion), recorded with a radio frequency locator system that also recorded the position of the biomagnetometer relative to the patient's head. MRI scans were obtained in the axial, sagittal, and coronal planes using a GE 1.5T Signa® scanner, with markers to show the preauricular points and nasion included on the scans to provide a common frame of reference to MEG. In some cases three-dimensional MRI acquisitions are combined with three-dimensional magnetic resonance angiograms to allow creation of a three-dimensional image of the head and blood vessels onto which the functional localizations can be projected. Such three-dimensional images were developed to aid neurosurgeons in visualizing functional brain maps to the brain surface features seen intra-operatively (14).

Of potential interest to the area of neurorehabilitation is the observation of slow wave sources localized at the margins of tissue affected by stroke, as visualized on MR (15). Observations with patients with chronic neurological signs due to head trauma have also shown MSI localizations of slow wave activity thought to be associated with white matter interruption (16).

Precise Functional Mapping of Sensory Evoked Fields

Auditory measurements using simple tones were the first to indicate a precise mapping of primary sensory cortical function. Pioneering studies with single channel biomagnetometers had revealed tonotopic map in the depth of Heschl's gyrus, with higher frequency tones being localized a few millimeters central to lower frequency tones in the depth of the gyrus (17,18). A later study with a large array biomagnetometer employed thirty repeated measures on the same subject, revealing maps for two separate "components" of the evoked waveforms occurring at about 90 and 170 msec. The two components were localized to sites separated by 8 mm within the primary

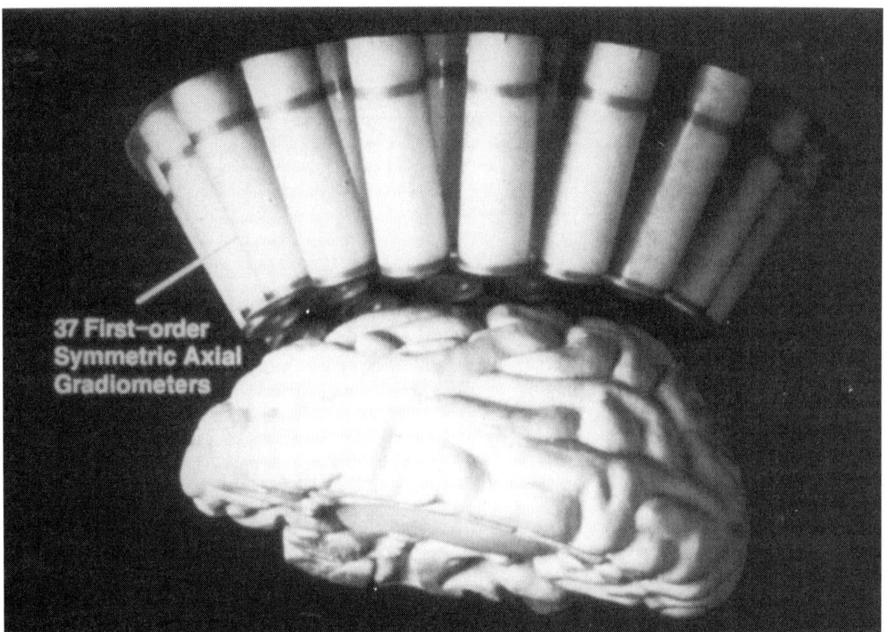

Figure 5-1. Layout of 37-channel Magnes® biomagnetometer axial gradiometer coils shown in relation to model brain of average size. (*Photo courtesy Biomagnetic Technologies, Inc., San Diego CA.*)

auditory cortex in Heschl's gyrus (19). The temporal and spatial resolving power of MSI was thus shown to be sufficient to track distinct sequences of events occurring within distances of millimeters and within latencies of several milliseconds. Such measurements established the experimental capacity of MSI to monitor *in vivo* abnormalities in cognitive and perceptual functioning.

Somatosensory evoked fields were measured using a standard clinical MSI protocol for presurgical functional mapping at the Scripps Clinic and Research Foundation. The result was a mapping of part of the Penfield somatosensory homunculus along the strip of the post-central gyrus. A pneumatically driven tactile stimulator applied a brief (40 msec) pulse of pressure at a rate of 2/sec to the thumb or index finger on the hand contralateral to the measured hemisphere, or to the lower lip (20). Localizations using the single equivalent dipole model were fit to averaged waveforms of 256 to 1,024 repetitions, and a somatosensory component peaking in the 45–75 msec latency range was mapped onto primary sensory cortex (S1), overlapping the source of the N19/P21 electrical evoked response (21,22). In order to obtain statistics on the error of localization for somatosensory functional mapping, a set of eighty repeated somatosensory measures was taken for a single stimulus site on one volunteer subject. Localizations were found to have a point-to-point standard deviation of 5.8 mm, with all localizations falling in the S1 area, posterior to the central sulcus (23).

Massive Cortical Reorganization Following Limb Amputation in Humans

Following the development of a clinical somatosensory measurement protocol for planning surgeries for tumor and epilepsy, a series of sensory evoked experiments was run on normal subjects in order to explore the spatial precision and accuracy of MSI-based localizations with respect to known physiological landmarks in normal human subjects seen on MR scans. The clinical protocol for somatosensory measurements had been limited to three stimulation sites on the hand and one site on the lower lip, each on the contralateral side to the hemisphere recorded with MEG. This was done in the interest of reducing measurement time and minimizing the discomfort of presurgical patients. For research volunteers, however, the number of measurements could be expanded considerably, so a set of measurements was undertaken to map out in fine detail the part of the homunculus extending from the hand to the upper arm and covering much of the face. Four neurologically normal volunteers were measured with the pneumatic stimulators applied to a total of sixty-six sites on the face, arm, and hand on each side of the body. MSI measurements showed distinct separations between locations representing discrete sites on the face and hand, and replicated the classical Penfield homunculus derived from surgical evoked measurements: areas enervating the lower arm and hand lie superior and medial to areas that map onto the face, and inferior and lateral to areas that map onto the upper arm and shoulder (24). There was clear spatial resolution of localizations representing closely spaced tactile sites on the hand and face. A complete map could be obtained in several 2–3 hour measurement sessions using the 37-channel biomagnetometer, a manageable time scale for measurements on amputee patients (25).

The impetus to this measurement was an opportunity to measure a set of four patients who had suffered accidental arm amputations at times ranging from five to forty-eight years in the past. These patients were being studied at UCSD by V. Ramachandran, who found that light touch or deep pressure to points on the face and the upper arm of the patients repeatedly and reliably evoked precisely localized referred sensations (RS) in their phantom limb. The small regions of skin that produced RS could be mapped onto specific areas of the limb, such as the digits. These points formed two clusters, one on the same side of the face as the phantom limb, and another near the line of amputation on the affected limb. The referred sensations proved to be modality specific, so that a drop of water trickling down the face would also be felt as a drop of water progressing along the phantom arm and fingers (26). This finding was suggestive of research on deafferented adult primates, where it was observed that cells originally receiving input from the arm later received input from the face, implying a cortical reorganization of a magnitude that extended far beyond the projection zones of single thalamocortical neurons (27).

Each of the four amputee patients was measured on a modified version of the experiment conducted with the four normals. The same sites were stimulated on both sides of the body except, of course, for the missing limb, but additionally facial sites that specifically gave rise to referred sensations were added, and the mirror image locations of these sites were stimulated on the contralateral side of the face. Also, when the patient reported a referred sensation on a particular spot on the phantom limb, the same spot on the unaffected contralateral hand was mapped.

The results indicated a large and dramatic cortical reorganization for the affected hemisphere of amputees. The maps of normals showed bilateral symmetry and mapped in the same ordinal way across subjects, as did the unaffected hemispheres on each of the amputee patients. By contrast, the maps of the affected hemispheres showed that localizations from face area occupied positions displaced in the direction and over-lapping the area presumably vacated by the hand, and occupied by the homologous hand area on the contralateral hemisphere. One case in point involved a patient who had suffered an accidental amputation of the right arm 8 cm below the elbow eleven years prior to examination with MSI (Figure 5-2). Facial sites producing referred sensations for this patient were displaced by 25–30 mm, while facial sites not producing RS were displaced 7–13 mm. Upper arm locations were also displaced by 10–20 mm toward the abandoned hand, invading from its territory superior and posterior (28). The same basic pattern of reorganization was seen on all three of the other amputees. In a more recent MSI study in a different laboratory, a larger sample (N = 13) of amputees with phantom limb pain were measured, and results showed a strong correlation between the extent of cortical remapping and the intensity of reported phantom limb pain, as measured on a standardized scale (29).

The cortical distances involved in these amputation studies imply neural remapping of connections far beyond the direct synaptic connections of thalamocortical afferents that may have survived the injury. One leading issue to address is the time course needed for cortical remapping to occur and whether this time course correlates strongly with recovery of function. Research on primates suggests that dramatic remapping may be very rapid and may even be reversible (30). Studies are underway in our labs to determine if repeated overstimulation can trigger changes in cortical maps detectable with MSI. In addition to the effects of nonstimulation, research with the auditory system of primates has suggested that cortical maps may be altered by selective and repeated "overstimulation" (31). The conjecture has been made that an assay of plasticity can be made for different patients and for different regions of cortex to help guide physical therapy or to help target pharmaceutical agents such as tissue plasminogen activators. A combination of reversible nerve blocks and overstimulation may provide for a rapid assay of cortical plasticity using functional imaging techniques including MSI.

For the present, in some cases, immediate relief from a phantom limb itch or pain may be provided by the patient's simply learning to scratch or rub the area of referred sensation. In the future, therapeutic relief from phantom limb pain may come with more understanding of the course of cortical remapping, along with the development of new rehabilitation procedures and pharmaceuticals, or even techniques of direct cortical stimulation.

Cortical Plasticity Due to Stroke: Preliminary Findings

Given that external injury can trigger a remapping of cortical areas, perhaps remapping may accompany deafferentation due to head trauma, stroke, or surgery to remove a tumor or epileptogenic site. Exploratory studies were conducted at the Scripps Clinic

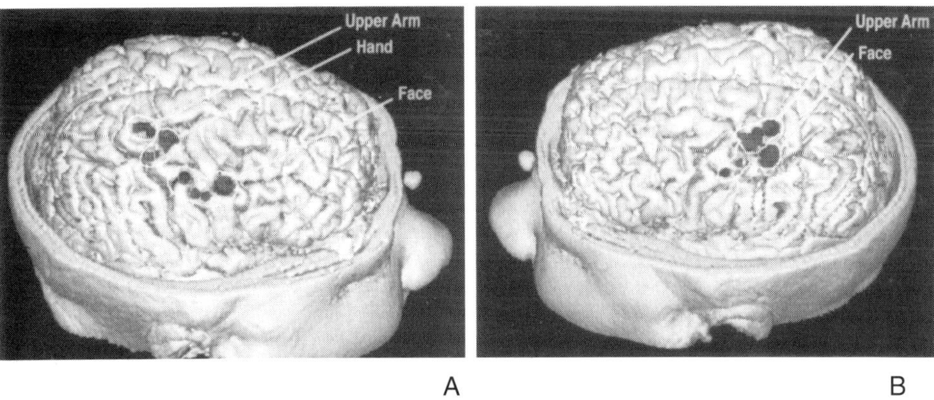

Figure 5-2. Three-dimensional volume renderings from MRI for the (A) unaffected (right) hemisphere and (B) affected (left) hemisphere for a 42-year-old male, studied eleven years after accidental amputation of his right arm 8 cm below the elbow. Psychophysical testing with light touch had revealed two separate "maps" of referred sensation (RS), with points referring to the phantom hand topographically organized and modality specific. One map was found on the upper right arm, above the stump, and a separate map was found on the right side of face extending along his chin, lower jaw, and cheek. MSI somatosensory localizations are shown projected onto the surface of the three-dimensional rendering. The unaffected (right) hemisphere shows a normal looking sequence of somatosensory localizations, with face, hand, and upper arm regions arrayed on a line moving from anterior, lateral, and inferior to posterior, medial, and superior locations. By contrast, the affected (left) hemisphere shows a map with facial sites moved in posterior, medial, and superior hand sites, and the upper arm sites having moved anterior, lateral, and inferior, so as to occupy the region homologous to the hand area on the contralateral hemisphere, presumed to have been vacated by afferent stimulation from the missing hand and lower arm. The three facial MSI locations producing RS were displaced by 25–30 mm as compared with the three facial sites not producing RS, which were displaced by 7–13 mm. All displacements were into the region.

and Research Foundation with twenty-five patients who had suffered massive strokes affecting the middle cerebral artery including primary somatosensory and motor cortex unilaterally. Many such patients were hemiplegic, did not feel the somatosensory stimuli, and produced no somatosensory evoked waveform that could be mapped at all, while others had impaired sensation and movement and generated weak but definite somatosensory responses. Four of the patients who had had some recovery of motor function and somatosensory sensation on the affected side also showed evidence of remapping of the somatosensory localizations of the affected side (32). These patients were found to have asymmetries in the localizations of the somatosensory evoked components, with dipoles from the unaffected hemisphere mapping onto the post-central gyrus, and dipoles from the affected side mapping as much as several centimeters posteriorly, beyond the margin of infarcted tissue as visualized on MR slices (Figure 5-3).

Although only five cases have been uncovered with apparent cortical displacement of somatosensory function, and data must be considered anecdotal, one interesting common denominator of all five cases may be worthy of mention. The remapped functional localizations have all moved to posterior sites, not to anterior sites, so that none moved across the central sulcus or into the frontal lobes. Perhaps more research will reveal a plasticity barrier line separating regions of afferent sensory functions from efferent (motor) areas. This hypothesis is supported in a limited way by the maps from our amputee subjects, where up to a 3 cm change in functional localizations still remained within the somatosensory strip and did not invade areas of motor cortex that had also been functionally abandoned.

Ongoing Developments of MSI Related to Neurorehabilitation

It may be expected that injury and rehabilitation will be accompanied by specific changes in both location and temporal patterns of neural regions mediating sensory and motor functions and cognitive processing. In this regard, MSI measurements of rhythmic cortical activity promise to open new ways of assessing functional cortical events associated with cognitive processes and cognitive deficits (33–35). The spatial and temporal precision of MSI makes it suitable for identifying and localizing changes in distribution of such rhythmic signals, as well as the more conventional averaged evoked responses. In the auditory modality, for example, the presence of a 40 Hz response following sensory stimulation, thought to be implicated in associating features from separate areas of cortex, has been mapped by MSI to the primary auditory cortex (36–38). It is also possible to measure and map difference waves using MSI, as, for example, in an auditory evoked study in which the primary 100 msec auditory magnetic response to tones of 1000 Hz and deviant tones of 1050 Hz were mapped. Using the single dipole model, the difference wave was localized significantly anterior, medial, and inferior relative to the sources of the M100, suggesting that a perceivable frequency deviation too small to activate measurably different dipoles may still access the nearby but spatially distinct mismatch generators (39). This kind of result suggests one way in which MSI can be used to track cortical changes accompanying auditory or somatosensory loss and recovery of capacity for making perceptual discriminations. Application to the realm of language processing would seem to be a high priority for neurorehabilitation.

Conclusions

Magnetic source imaging can add significantly to methods of functional imaging such as PET and fMRI, which can map central structures related to processing tasks, but which are limited in spatial and temporal resolution by the speed of metabolic processes or the reaction time for blood oxygenation (40). The advantage of MSI lies in its capacity for measurement of regional neural events directly. More of the full potential of MSI will be seen with the continued development of whole head MSI systems (see Figure 5-3) capable of detecting sources at greater depths from the surface (41). Also, more advanced methods of modeling source activity will transcend the single dipole model used to map evoked responses. The mapping of evoked and spon-

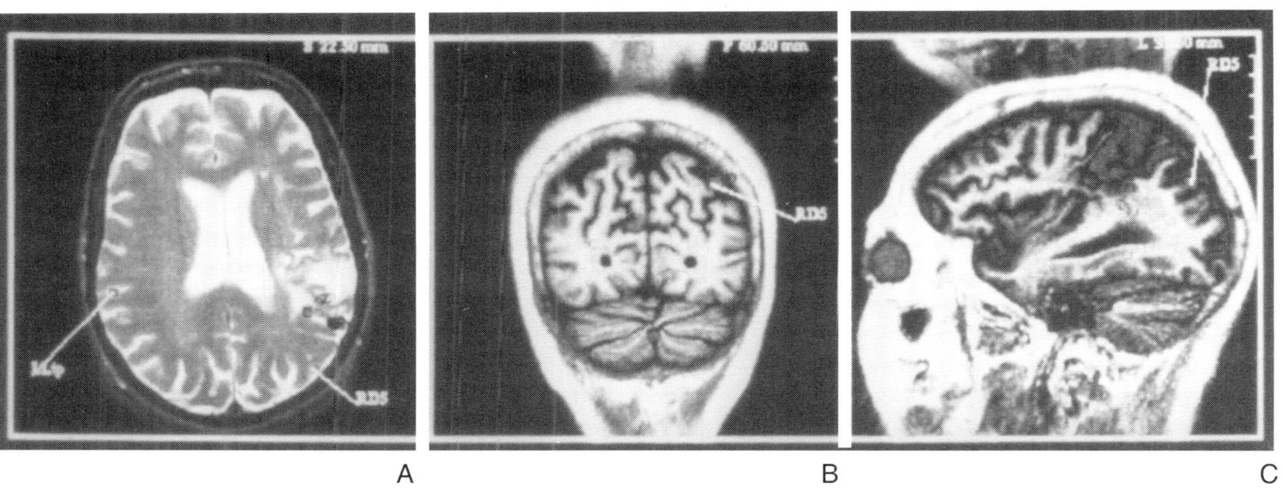

Figure 5-3. MSI overlay showing somatosensory localizations in (A) axial, (B) coronal, and (C) sagittal MR slices for a 73-year-old woman who had suffered a middle cerebral arterial stroke on the left hemisphere, with a completed cerebral infarction mostly affecting the left parietal lobe. Slow wave MSI dipole localizations (*dark squares*) can be seen in the axial slice in the posterior margin of the infarcted area. A functional somatosensory MSI localization from the right fifth digit localized more than 2 cm posterior to the central sulcus on the affected slice. In comparison, a localization from facial stimulation (LLip), which localized to the same axial slice on the unaffected right hemisphere, appears in the region of the post-central gyrus, as expected. Partial recovery of motor function and somatosensory sensitivity had been noted on the patient's affected side.

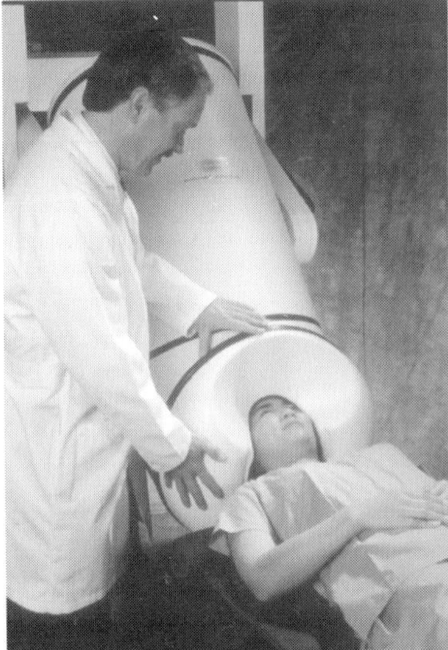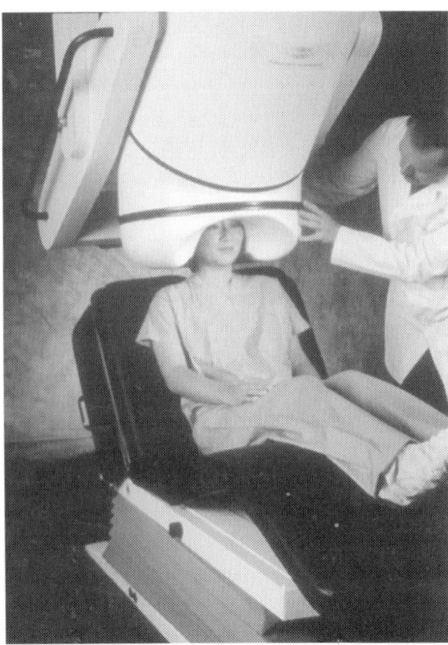

Figure 5-4. A 148-channel whole head biomagnetometer system shown for use with reclining or seated patients. (*Photo courtesy Biomagnetic Technologies, Inc., San Diego CA.*)

taneous signals promises to be advanced significantly with models that combine structural information on cortical geometry with MEG and EEG data in order to map multiple sources and more extended neural sources (42–44).

Acknowledgments: This work was supported by the Armstrong McDonald Foundation, the McDonnell-PEW Foundation, the Pasarow Foundation, and by a cooperative agreement with Biomagnetic Technologies, Inc.

References

1. Gallen CC, Sobel DF, Lewine JD, et al. Neuromagnetic mapping of brain function. *Radiology* 1993;187(3):863–67.
2. Gallen CC, Pantev C, Hampson S, Buchanan DS, Sobel DF. Reliability and validity of auditory neuromagnetic source localizations using a large array biomagnetometer. In: Hoke M, Erne SN, Okada Y, Romani GL (eds.). *Biomagnetism: clinical aspects.* Proceedings of the 8th International Conference on Biomagnetism. Amsterdam: Elsevier Science Publishers, 1992:171–75.
3. Williamson SJ, Kaufman L (1987) Analysis of neuromagnetic signals. In: Gevins A, Remond A (eds.). *Handbook of electroencephalography and clinical neurophysiology* (revised series, Vol. 1). Amsterdam: Elsevier, 1987:405–48.
4. Okada Y. Physiological basis of magnetoencephalography. *Biomed Eng*1986;14:84.
5. Kaufman L, Williamson SJ. The neuromagnetic field. In: Cracco RQ, Bodis-Wolner (eds.). *Evoked potentials: frontiers of clinical science.* New York: Alan R. Liss, 1986:85–98.
6. Vieth J, Grummich P, Sack G, et al. Three-dimensional localization of the pathological area in cerebro-vascular accidents with multichannel magnetoencephalography *Biomed Eng* 1990; 35(Suppl 2):238–39.

7. Gallen CC, Sobel DF, Waltz T, et al. Noninvasive presurgical neuromagnetic mapping of somatosensory cortex. *Neurosurgery* 1993;33(2):260–68.

8. Eisenberg HM, Papanicolaou AC, et al. Magnetoencephalographic localization of inter-ictal spike sources: case report. *J Neurosurg* 1991;74:660–64.

9. Sutherling WW, Crandall PH, Cahan LD, Barth DS. The magnetic field of epileptic spikes agrees with intracranial localizations in complex partial epilepsy. *Neurology* 1988;38(5):778–86.

10. Paetau R, Hämäläinen R, Hari R, et al. Magnetoencephalographic evaluation of children and adolescents with intractable epilepsy. *Epilepsia* 1994;35(2):275–84.

11. Sobel DF, Gallen CC, Schwartz BJ, et al. Locating the central sulcus: comparison of MR anatomic and magnetoencephalographic functional methods. *Am J Neuroradiology* 1993;14:915–25.

12. Gallen CC, Bucholz R, Sobel DF. Intracranial neurosurgery guided by functional imaging. *Surgical Neurology* 1994;42:523–30.

13. Gallen CC, Schwartz BJ, Bucholz R, et al. Presurgical localization of functional cortex using magnetic source imaging. *J Neurosurg* 1995;82:988–94.

14. Gallen CC, Sobel DF, Waltz T, et al. Noninvasive pre-surgical neuromagnetic mapping of somatosensory cortex. *Neurosurgery* 1993;33(2):260–68.

15. Gallen C, Schwartz BJ, Pantev C, et al. Detection and localization of delta frequency activity in human strokes. In: Hoke M, Erne SN, Okada Y, Romani GL (eds.). *Biomagnetism: clinical aspects.* Proceedings of the 8th International Conference on Biomagnetism. Amsterdam: Elsevier Science Publishers, 1992:301–305.

16. Schwartz BJ, Aung A, Gallen CC, Sobel DF, Hirschkoff EC, Bloom FE. Magnetoencephalographic detection of focal slowing associated with head trauma. *Proceedings of the 9th International Conference on Biomagnetism.* Amsterdam: Elsevier Science, 1994 (in press).

17. Romani GL, Williamson SJ, Kaufman L. Tonotopic organization of the human auditory cortex. *Science* 1982;216:1339–40.

18. Pantev C, Lehnertz K, Lütkenhöner B, Anogianakis G, Wittkowski W. Tonotopic organization of the human auditory cortex revealed by transient auditory evoked magnetic fields. *Electroenceph Clin Neurophysiol* 1988;69:160–70.

19. Pantev C, Gallen C, Hampson S, Buchanan S, Sobel D. Reproducibility and validity of neuromagnetic source localization using a large array biomagnetometer. *Am J EEG Technol* 1991;31:83–101.

20. Schwartz BJ, Gallen CC, Hampson S, Hirschkoff EC, Sobel DF, Rieke K. Reliability of somatosensory neuromagnetic source localizations using a Multisensor Biomagnetometer. In: Hoke M, Erne SN, Okada Y, Romani GL (eds.). *Biomagnetism: clinical aspects.* Proceedings of the 8th International Conference on Biomagnetism. Amsterdam: Elsevier Science Publishers, 1992:253–57.

21. Hari R, Kaukoranta E. Neuromagnetic studies of somatosensory system: principles and examples. *Progress in Neurobiology* 1985;24:233–56.

22. Hari R, Reinikainen K, Kaukoranta E, et al. Somatosensory evoked cerebral magnetic fields from SI and SII in man. *Electroenceph Clin Neurophysiol* 1984;57:254–63.

23. Gallen CC, Schwartz BJ, Rieke K, et al. Intrasubject reliability and validity of somatosensory source localization using a large array biomagnetometer. *J Electroencephalog Clin Neurophysiolol* 1994;90(2):145–56.

24. Yang TT, Gallen CC, Schwartz BJ, Bloom FE. Noninvasive somatosensory homunculus mapping in humans by using a large-array biomagnetometer. *Proc Nat Acad Sciences* 1993;90:3098–3102.

25. Yang TT, Gallen, CC, Ramachandran, VS, Cobb S, Schwartz BJ, Bloom FE. Noninvasive detection of cerebral plasticity in adult human somatosensory cortex. *NeuroReports* 1994;5(6):701–704.

26. Ramachandran VS, Rogers-Ramachandran D, Stewart M. Perceptual correlates of massive cortical reorganization. *Science* 1992;258:1159–60.

27. Pons TP, Garraghty PE, Ommaya AK, Kaas JH, Taub E, Mishkin M. Massive cortical reorganization after sensory deafferentation in adult macaques. *Science* 1991;252:1857–60.
28. Yang TT, Gallen CC, Ramachandran V, Cobb SJ, Bloom FE, Schwartz BJ. Sensory maps in the human brain, *Nature* 1994;368(14): 592–93.
29. Flor H, Elbert T, Knecht S, et al. Phantom-limb pain as a perceptual correlate of cortical reorganization following arm amputation. *Nature* 1995;375:482–84.
30. Recanzone GH, Merzenich MM, Schreiner CE. Changes in the distributed temporal response properties of SI cortical neurons reflect improvements in performance on a temporally based tactile discrimination task. *J Neurophysiol* 1992;67(5):1071–91.
31. Recanzone GH, Schreiner CE, Merzenich MM. Plasticity in the frequency representation of primary auditory cortex following discrimination training in adult owl monkeys. *J Neurosci* 1993;13(1):87–103.
32. Rieke K, Gallen CC, Sobel DF, et al. Magnetic source localization somatosensory cortex in stroke: evidence for cerebral plasticity. Proceedings, American Society of Neuroradiology (ASNR) 31st Annual Meeting, May 16–20, 1993. Vancouver, BC, Canada. Paper #139, p. 104.
33. Salmelin R, Hari R. Characterization of spontaneous MEG rhythms in healthy adults. *Electroenceph Clin Neurophysiol* 1994;91:237–48.
34. Kaufman L, Schwartz BJ, Salustri C, Williamson SJ. Modulation of spontaneous brain activity. *J Cognitive Neuroscience* 1990;2:124–32
35. Gallen CC, Hampson S, Young W, Bloom FE. Reactivity of neuromagnetic alpha frequency activity in human subjects. *Society for Neuroscience Abstracts* 1989;15(1): 121 (Ab. 53.4).
36. Ribary U, Ioannides AA, Singh KD, et al. Magnetic field tomography (MFT) of coherent thalamo-cortical 40 Hz oscillations in humans. *Proc Nat Acad Sci (USA)* 1991 88:11037–41.
37. Singer W, Gray CM, Engel A, Konig P, Artola A, Brocher S. Formation of cortical cell assemblies. *Cold Spring Harbor Symposia on Quantitative Biology* 1990;55:939–53.
38. Hari R, Mäkelä JP. Evidence for cortical origin of the 40 Hz auditory evoked response in man. *Electroenceph Clin Neurophysiol* 1987;66: 539–46.
39. Csepe V, Pantev C, Hoke M, Hampson S, Ross B. Evoked magnetic responses of the human auditory cortex to minor pitch changes: localization of the mismatch field. *Electroencephal Clin Neurophysiol* 1992;84(6):538–48.
40. Kwong KK, Belliveau JW, Chesler DA, et al. Dynamic magnetic resonance imaging of human brain activity during primary sensory stimulation. *Proc Nat Acad Sciences* (USA) 1992;89(12):5675–79.
41. Lounasmaa OV, Knuutila J, Salmelin R. SQUID technology and brain research. *Physica B* 1994;197:54–63.
42. Dale AM, Sereno MI. Improved localization of cortical activity by combining EEG and MEG with MRI cortical surface reconstruction: a linear approach. *J Cognitive Neuroscience* 1993;5(2):162–76.
43. Ioannides A, Fenwick PB, Lumsden J, et al. Activation sequence of discrete brain areas during cognitive processes: results from magnetic field tomography. *Electroenceph Clin Neurophysiol* 1994;91(5):399–402.
44. Wang JZ, Williamson SJ, Kaufman L. Magnetic source imaging based on the minimum-norm least-squares inverse [review]. *Brain Topography* 1993;5(4):365–71.

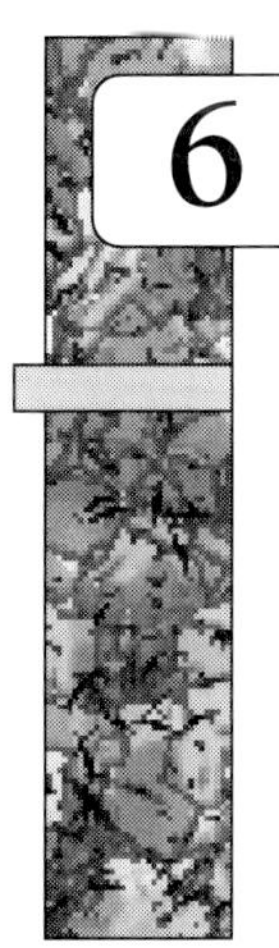

6

The Relationship Between Functional Assessment and Outcome

Roger C. Fiedler, **Ph.D.**, and
Carl V. Granger, **M.D.**

Functional assessment is a method for describing the abilities and limitations an individual experiences in order to measure the performance of the activities that are necessary to daily living. However, functional assessment may also be used to model the expected progress of a person who has a disability. It may be assumed that people who experience disability are relatively intact before an illness, stroke, or accident causes them to lose function in these activities. Although they have been diagnosed and stabilized in acute care, they typically have not recovered sufficient function to return home. It is expected that a rehabilitation program will rebuild their function, perhaps not to where they were, but to a point that is suitable for functioning in the community.

Figure 6-1 shows that when level of function is measured on rehabilitation admission, it is expected that improvement toward more independence in the basic activities will occur over time. In Figure 6-1, the vertical distance between status on admission and that at discharge represents the effectiveness of the program in a measurable way. This number divided by the length of stay in days represents the gain per day or the efficiency of the functional gain. About fourteen years ago, thirteen national rehabilitation organizations supported a program to develop a standard way of describing disability and the outcomes of rehabilitation. This was called the Uniform Data System for Medical Rehabilitation (UDSmr[SM]) (1). The functional assessment instrument incorporated into the UDSmr[SM] is the Functional Independence Measure (FIM[SM] instrument). The major goals of medical rehabilitation are to improve level of functional performance by raising the FIM score and to provide the severely disabled person with sufficient function to have improved options for restoring that person's quality of daily living. Quality of Daily Living is distinguished from quality of life in that it reflects the functional nature of daily living, and may be operationally defined as follows:

Quality of Daily Living is the ever-changing balance between one's choices, options, and expectations versus the physical, cognitive, and emotional demands of daily living.

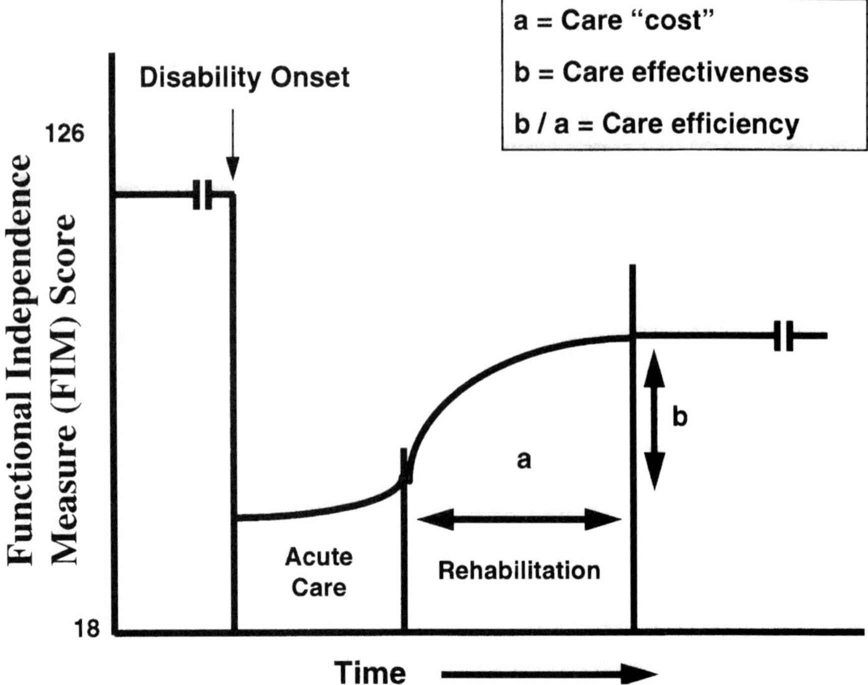

Figure 6-1. The relationship between effectiveness and efficiency in medical rehabilitation.

This operational definition is represented in Figure 6-2, which indicates that fulfillment in daily living results from creating a balance in life between the functional opportunities available to the individual on the one hand, with the functional requirements or demands placed on the individual on the other. Thus, Figure 6-2 not only represents a conceptual way to achieve Quality of Daily Living but also allows for the operational measurement of the factors that determine opportunities and requirements (demands) using a variety of scales including functional assessment scales. Figure 6-2 represents an entirely new organizing and unifying model for studying disability and outcomes in medical rehabilitation. This model focuses on a new conceptual framework of Challenges to the Quality of Daily Living and covers a broad range of concerns currently under debate in the field of medical rehabilitation.

The Challenges to Quality of Daily Living model develops from the work of the noted American psychologist Abraham Maslow. Maslow (2) advanced a new theory of human motivation that challenged some of the orthodox principles of Freudian and Skinnerian psychology. Prior to Maslow, it had been considered appropriate to control and manipulate employees in the workplace. In the 1960s, Maslow developed the "Eupsychian Management" way of thinking to encourage a more humanistic relationship between management and employees. From this, Maslow evolved a hierarchy of needs that would support self-actualization. At the base of his conceptual pyramid lay the physical needs for survival. At progressively higher levels

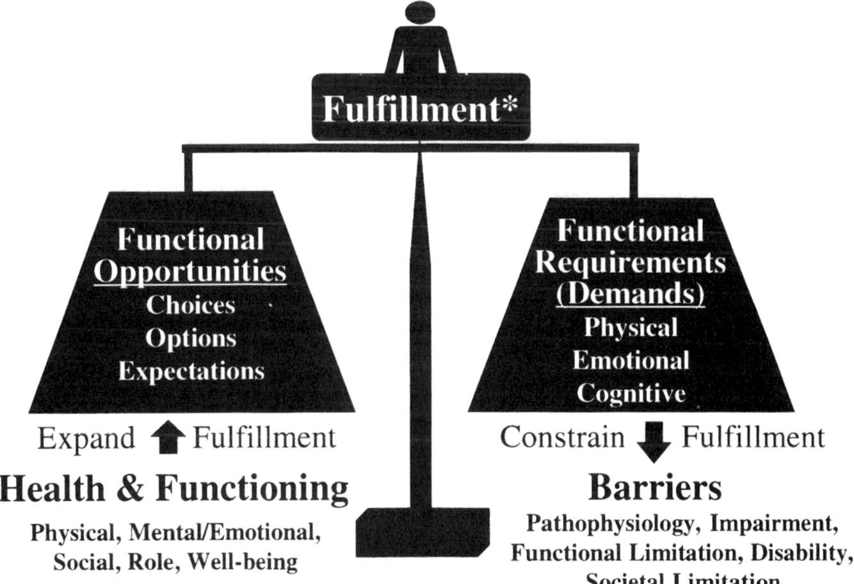

Figure 6-2. Challenges to Quality of Daily Living.

were satisfaction of needs for security, social interaction, and self-esteem. As lower level needs were satisfied, then successively higher levels of need became relatively more important as motivators of behavior. Ultimately, the fully evolved individual would achieve self-actualization, a term that describes the full utilization of human capacities to perceive, feel, learn, acquire skills, exercise intellectual capabilities, create, love—in short, based on self-esteem and respect for others, to grow in competence and ability to live a fulfilling life (2).

Maslow's concepts form the conceptual framework for the study of disability outcomes. Medical rehabilitation is a system of interdisciplinary interventions designed to facilitate fulfillment and the quality of daily living for individuals with disabilities. Medical rehabilitation needs measurement that can reflect effectiveness and efficiency of the process. Yet to a large extent, fulfillment and quality of daily living are not directly measurable. However, in order to account for the challenges to fulfillment and the quality of daily living, one must begin by identifying the factors that determine the opportunities and requirements (demands). Figure 6-2 proposes that an individual's fulfillment and quality of daily living are the result of striking a balance between functional opportunities (on the left) and functional requirements or demands (on the right). Functional opportunities are expressed as the individual's choices, options, and expectations, while functional requirements are expressed in physical, cognitive, and emotional terms. In order to achieve fulfillment and to maximize the quality of daily living, there must be a balance between improved opportunities through individual health and functioning (on the left) and the reduction or removal of life's barriers causing constraints (on the right). This model reflects Maslow's industrial psychological beliefs that health and functioning result from the individual's being presented with life's work in the form of barriers and systematically overcoming them. The model further reflects Maslow's hierarchical beliefs in that it views the individual with a disability as meeting progressively higher needs of function through the work of medical rehabilitation. The field of medical rehabilitation recognizes the need for balance between functional demands and functional opportunities, progressively presenting both the demands and the ways to achieve the opportunities to the patient in the form of challenges to the quality of daily living, and moving up the hierarchy from the basic physical needs to the satisfaction for security, social interaction, and self-esteem. The ultimate goal of medical rehabilitation then becomes, in Maslow's terms, self-actualization, the full utilization of the human capacities to perceive, feel, create, and love, in the form of fulfillment through the everyday efforts to challenge barriers and overcome them.

Figure 6-2 includes several measurable factors that serve as domains of health and functioning (on the left) such as physical, mental/emotional, social, role performance, and subjective well-being, while measurable barriers (on the right) include pathophysiology, impairment, functional limitation, disability, and societal limitation.

This unifying model for medical rehabilitation fits well with existing theoretical frameworks across the many disciplines involved in medical rehabilitation [e.g., the Open Systems Theory Models of von Bertalanffy (3) and Kielhofner & Burke (4)] of hierarchical structures and expanding and constraining relationships between levels of the hierarchy, and provides an organizing conceptual framework for measuring disability across disciplines in medical rehabilitation. The model recognizes that functional opportunities and requirements that serve as the Challenges to the Quality of Daily Living are not directly measurable, but that the factors that determine the opportunities and requirements are subject to description and measurement.

The model of Challenges to the Quality of Daily Living represented in Figure 6-2 suggests that fulfillment results from a balance between the functional opportunities to expand health and functioning through choices, options, and expectations, while at the same time overcoming the challenges of functional barriers in the form of physical, emotional, and cognitive demands that constrain function. It is clear that the examination of such complexity is not easily achieved through current medical rehabilitation measures. However, the factors that determine the opportunities and requirements or demands are subject to description and measurement. One of the goals of developing such a model is to translate the concepts into measurement systems, and then to implement those systems into clinical practice through research.

In order to determine how well a conceptual theoretical model fits the field of medical rehabilitation, the model must be judged on its comprehensiveness, its ability to be subject to the principles of good measurement, and its practicality in implementation. And it must be rigorously tested by patients, clinicians, and administrators, as well as by researchers in the literature.

The model proposed in Figure 6-2 is quite comprehensive, as it allows for the inclusion of a multidisciplinary approach to the field of medical rehabilitation. The process of translating the model into measurement and the practicality of implementing it into the clinical arena where it may be judged by patients, clinicians, and the like has begun with the use of the Functional Independence Measure (FIM) at the Uniform Data System for Medical Rehabilitation (UDSMR^{SM}) at the State University of New York at Buffalo. The UDSMR^{SM} is not only a data repository and reporting system, but includes important feedback loops, system supports, training, credentialing, and research.

The initial development of the FIM instrument involved concerns for validity, reliability, feasibility, and precision. The interrater reliability was studied on 1,018 inpatients in 89 hospitals using intraclass correlation coefficients (ICCs) and kappa statistics for individual FIM items (5). The ICC for the total FIM was .96, which was acceptable. The lowest subscale ICC was .89 for social cognition. The kappa statistics for the 18 items ranged from .53 to .66, which was also acceptable. The underlying concept for developing the FIM was to produce a metric that would reflect need for assistance or a measurement of the burden of care. To investigate this, three groups of patients were evaluated at home—multiple sclerosis, stroke, and spinal cord injury, using the FIM. Caregivers in the home were instructed to use a stopwatch to measure the minutes of assistance that they provided to the subject. Regression analysis showed that 77% of the variance between FIM scores and minutes of help was explained in subjects with multiple sclerosis (6), 65% for stroke (7), and 76% for spinal cord injury (8). One FIM point was equivalent to 3–5 minutes of help from another person. Thus, this instrument aids the clinician in estimating the burden of care of patients with severe disability.

The next move was to develop a uniform database from the data submitted by subscribing facilities from admission, discharge, and follow-up records. In the first full year, 1988, there were 33,000 records reported to the UDSMR^{SM}, which increased to 127,000 records in 1993 (9,10). The rehabilitation patients are identified by impairment group. In 1990 there were 11,000 stroke cases, 15,000 in 1991, 26,000 in 1992, and 40,000 in 1993. Stroke comprises about one-third of the total caseload. Fewer than half of the stroke cases are males, the mean age has remained about 70–71, and the days between onset and admission to rehabilitation has dropped from 22 to 19. Admission and discharge mean total FIM scores have remained stable at about 62 and 87, respectively. Efficiency, reflected as FIM gain per week, has been increasing from 5.4 points to 6.4 points. This is associated with a drop in length of stay from 32 days to 26 days. Thus, length of stay has been decreasing despite rather constant values in admission severity and gain in FIM points to discharge (9,10).

Looking at the relationship between side of paresis, age, and length of acute and rehabilitation stay for all types of stroke patients, those under the age of 65 had the longest total hospital stays while patients aged 80 years or older had the shortest stays, in both acute and rehabilitative care. Patients with bilateral hemiparesis (about 4% of the group) had longer stays than those with left or right hemiparesis, under age 80 but with little difference over age 80 (11).

Stroke patients with bilateral hemiparesis and age 80 years or older were more disabled on admission and made less gain than unilateral patients and patients under age 80. In motor functions governing self-care, sphincter management, transferring, and locomotion, the FIM scores were the same for right and left at admission and discharge. The differences in communication and social cognition were as expected. Patients with left hemiparesis without aphasia had higher admission and discharge scores in both communication and social cognition than patients with right hemiparesis and left hemisphere lesions (11).

The discharge FIM score is related to the expectation of a patient being discharged to the community. For example, if a program sets a goal of returning 75–77% of patients with stroke to the community, then one would expect that group of patients to have an average discharge total FIM score of 80. Based on studies of stroke and other patients at home (6,7), we learned that within the range of 55 to 115 total FIM scores, one FIM point is worth about 3–5 minutes of help per day from another person. Combining the two pieces of information, we see that a target discharge score of 80 corresponds to about two hours of help per day. Thus, a patient who is discharged home with a total FIM score below 80 will require more than two hours of assistance per day, a burden of care that may not be manageable by the family. Patients with scores higher than 80 will require less than two hours of help, a level that seems to be tolerable in most family situations.

If a discharge FIM score of 80 is a reasonable level for return to the community, then the next question is to what extent is this proportion affected by other patient factors? Regarding age, the proportion of patients discharged to the community is higher with younger patients; 83% for patients under 65 years old, 75% for patients 65 to 79 years old, and 64% for patients 80 years old and over (11). However, of those patients who were discharged to the community, older patients are more likely to have FIM scores below 80 than are the younger patients. Of patients living alone, more were likely to have FIM scores over 80. This is understandable as patients living alone would need to be more independent than patients who live with others. Having left or right hemiparesis did not affect the proportion of patients discharged to the community with discharge FIM scores over or under 80. However, a slightly larger percent of bilaterally affected patients had different rates of discharge to the community based on male or female gender. However, a slightly greater proportion of black than white patients had discharge FIM scores below 80.

Being able to predict which patients will reside in the community six months after completion of a rehabilitation program would be intriguing. In a multicenter study of ten facilities and 539 stroke patients (12), the predictive ability of knowing the patient's independent versus dependent performance in four ADL functions was studied. The rehabilitation admission status, on average three weeks after acute onset, of eating, grooming, bladder control, and bowel control was studied. Table 6-1 shows the results of determining who was living in the community at six–month follow-up based on number of items at admission in which patients were independent in the four functions of eating, bowel control, bladder control, and grooming.

It was determined that the best cut point for identifying who was likely to be living in the community at six-month follow-up based on Independence vs. Dependence at admission in the four functions of eating, bowel control, bladder control, and grooming was zero to one vs. two or more with a 66% probability [least mean error (13) of 34%].

Table 6-1. *Patient status at 6-month follow-up as a function of 4-function independence at admission.* *

	Patient Status at 6-Month Follow-up		
Independence in Combined Functions of: 1—Eating 2—Bowel 3—Bladder 4—Grooming	Living in Community	Living in LTCF[1] or Died	Totals
Two or More	234 (82%) (64%)	50 (18%) (29%)	284
Zero to One	133 (52%) (36%)	122 (48%) (71%)	255
Totals	367	172	539

*Percentages in parentheses represent row and column percentages.
[1]LTCF = long-term care facility.

Looking at Table 6-1 prospectively shows that of the patients who were independent in none or only one of the functions of eating, bowel control, bladder control, and grooming at admission to rehabilitation, 52% of them were living in the community six months after discharge. However, of the patients who were independent in two or more functions of eating, bowel control, bladder control, and grooming at admission to rehabilitation, 82% of them were living in the community six months after discharge.

Looking at Table 1 retrospectively shows that of the patients who were living in the community six months after discharge, 64% had been independent in two or more functions on admission to rehabilitation. Of the patients who were living in long-term care facilities or had died by six months after discharge, 72% had been independent in none or only one of the functions on admission to rehabilitation.

These individual patterns were examined using logistic regression prediction models adjusting for patient age, sex, and hemiparesis. Odds ratios computed from the logistic regression compared patients with independence in one or more functions to those without independence in any of the four functions at admission. The results showed that patients independent in one function, usually bowel, had a three times greater likelihood for residing in the community six months after rehabilitation discharge. Patients who were independent in bowel and eating, or bowel and grooming, had a six times greater likelihood of living in the community. Patients independent in bowel, eating, and grooming had eleven times greater likelihood of living in the community. Patients independent in all four items had fourteen times more likelihood of living in the community than patients who were dependent in the four items. Thus, the admission status to rehabilitation in terms of patients' independence in these very basic functions was a predictor of the likelihood of being in the community after completion of rehabilitation.

We have also investigated the measurement characteristics of the FIM instrument. The FIM was developed to be an ordinal scale where level 3 is greater than level 2 but the distance between the levels may not be the same as that between levels 4 and 5. Some authors (14) have raised the question of "misinferences" based on the practice of adding item scores together and making interpretations from total scores. The technique of Rasch analysis was used to construct interval measures from the ordinal FIM data (15). The Rasch modeling technique also constructs unidimensional measures by simultaneously measuring subjects and items on the same scale and analyzes the person–item interactions. The major factors taken into account are the relative difficulty in performance of test items and the ability of persons tested. What was discovered was that the FIM was composed of two measures, the first 13 items defining a motor dimension and the last 5 items defining a cognitive dimension, each with good measurement characteristics (16–20). Rasch analysis also defines how easy or hard the individual items are along a hierarchical continuum. Thus, of the motor items, eating is the easiest and stairclimbing is the hardest, and of the cognitive items, comprehension is the easiest and problem-solving is the hardest. With the understanding that is revealed through Rasch analysis, it is possible to use the raw motor or cognitive scores to estimate the probable scores of each of the items. One must keep in mind that different clinical entities have different expected patterns in terms of the hierarchy of items. For example, for the motor domain, orthopedic cases define a general hierarchical continuum that is similar to stroke except that dressing is relatively more difficult for stroke. Spinal cord dysfunction is different because of relatively more difficulty in controlling bladder and bowel. In the cognitive domain, expression is more difficult for right hemiparetic patients with aphasia, social interaction is more difficult for patients with severe spinal cord dysfunction (e.g., tetraplegia), and memory and problem-solving are more difficult for patients with brain dysfunction.

The most recent developments include technologic advances to improve accuracy of data, bringing the data closer to the clinicians, improving functional prognostication, and allowing rapid access to the facility's own data. This software program, called FIMware™, should facilitate communication among members of the team and more efficient achievement of patient care goals. A part of this facilitation is achieved through use of the FIM profile, which is a circular graph that depicts the patient's change in status over time. This report can be printed and incorporated into the patient's clinical record. In the FIM profile each of the 18 items is represented by a point on a series of concentric circles. The inner circle represents the lowest function at level 1 and the outer circle represents the highest function at level 7.

With the advent of managed care, it is imperative that rehabilitation facilities use a classification system that, on admission, projects the likely length of stay of a group of patients of similar type. Investigations by Dr. Margaret Stineman and her colleagues (21) have resulted in development of function related groups (Penn Ability Systems™ (PAS™)FIM=FRGs). The intent of FRGs was to provide a basis for a new prospective payment system for rehabilitation that is similar to the DRGs, in order to correct the inequities of the present TEFRA system. Under TEFRA the facility is paid the same for any discharge once the TEFRA limits have been specified. Older hospitals have a lower cost basis and are reimbursed much less than newer hospitals that have different cost basis for the same set of patients. Aside from being unfair, it imposes an incentive for facilities to avoid difficult patients who may consume a lot of resources in favor of treating patients who might require fewer resources and stay a shorter period of time in the hospital.

In order to be feasible, the system that predicts length of stay has to be simple and stable across a mixture of types of patients. The FIM-FRG system was developed using cases in the UDSmr^{SM} database between January 1, 1990, and March 31, 1991, based on first admissions for rehabilitation. Subjects were 16 years of age or older and length of stay was greater than 3 days but less than 1 year. Patients who died were excluded. Groups were clustered on the basis of type of impairment, such as stroke, brain injury, spinal cord injury, and so on. The admission FIM motor and cognitive scores plus age were used to develop the classification. The analysis produced 18 impairment groups (6 neurological, 7 musculoskeletal, and 5 miscellaneous), which are divided into 53 FIM-FRGs based on the logarithm of the length of stay. Fourteen percent of the variance was explained by just the diagnostic categories. By adding the functional scores and age, the amount of variance explained went up to 31%.

Residual needs in stroke rehabilitation research include determining how much improvement is due to spontaneous recovery and how much is due to the rehabilitation program. Function predicts function. Would addition of measures of impairment (similar to the NIH scale) enhance the prediction of function? In order to make study populations more homogeneous and comparable, studies should incorporate stratification techniques similar to those used to develop FIM-FRGs. The relationship between the employment of rehabilitation resources, including venue of service, and outcomes needs to be made more explicit.

References

1. Hamilton BB, Granger CV, Sherwin FS, Zielezny M, Tashman JS. A uniform national data system for medical rehabilitation. In: Fuhrer MJ (ed.). *Rehabilitation outcomes: analysis and measurement.* Baltimore: Brookes, 1987:137–47.
2. Maslow AH. *Motivation and personality.* New York: Harper & Row, 1954.
3. Von Bertalanffy L. *General system theory: foundations, development, applications.* New York: Braziller, 1968.
4. Kielhofner G, Burke JP. A model of human occupation. Part 1. Conceptual framework and content. *Am J Occ Ther* 1980;34(9):572–81.
5. Hamilton BB, Laughlin JL, Fiedler RC, Granger CV. Interrater reliability of the 7-level Functional Independence Measure (FIM). *Scand J Rehab Med* 1994;26:115–19.
6. Granger CV, Cotter AC, Hamilton BB, Fiedler RC. Functional assessment scales: a study of persons with multiple sclerosis. *Arch Phys Med Rehabil* 1990;71:870–75.
7. Granger CV, Cotter AC, Hamilton BB, Fiedler RC. Functional assessment scales: a study of persons after stroke. *Arch Phys Med Rehabil* 1993;74:133–38.
8. Hamilton BB, Granger CV. The cost of disability as measured by the Functional Independence Measure (FIM): spinal cord injury. Project H133A80002. National Institute on Disability and Rehabilitation Research, State University of New York at Buffalo, 1991.
9. Granger CV, Hamilton BB. UDS report: The Uniform Data System for Medical Rehabilitation report of the first admissions for 1990. *Am J Phys Med Rehabil* 1992;71:108–13.

10. Granger CV, Ottenbacher KJ, Fiedler RC. The Uniform Data System for Medical Rehabilitation report of first admissions for 1993. *Am J Phys Med Rehabil* 1995;74:62–66.

11. Granger CV, Hamilton BB, Fiedler RC. Discharge after stroke rehabilitation. *Stroke* 1992;23:978–82.

12. Granger CV, Hamilton BB, Gresham GE, Kramer AA. The stroke rehabilitation outcome study. Part II. Relative merits of the total Barthel Index score and a four-item subscore in predicting patient outcomes. *Arch Phys Med Rehabil* 1989;70:100–103.

13. Armitage P. *Statistical methods in medical research.* Boston: Halstead, 1971.

14. Merbitz C, Morris J, Grip JC. Ordinal scales and foundations of misinference. *Arch Phys Med Rehabil* 1989;70:308–12.

15. Wright BD, Linacre JM. *BIGSTEPS: a Rasch-model computer program.* Chicago: MESA Press, 1991.

16. Heinemann AW, Hamilton BB, Granger CV, Linacre JM, Wright BD. Rehabilitation efficacy for brain and spinal cord injury—final report. Project R49/CCR503609. Centers for Disease Control. Chicago: Rehabilitation Institute of Chicago, 1992.

17. Heinemann AW, Hamilton BB, Granger CV, Wright BD, Linacre JM. Final report: rating scale analysis of functional assessment measure. Project #133H90167: Department of Education, National Institute on Disability and Rehabilitation Research. Chicago: Rehabilitation Institute of Chicago, 1991.

18. Heinemann AW, Linacre JM, Wright BD, Hamilton BB, Granger CV. Relationships between impairment and disability as measured by the Functional Independence Measure. *Arch Phys Med Rehabil* 1993;74:566–73.

19. Heinemann AW, Linacre JM, Wright BD, Hamilton BB, Granger CV. Measurement characteristics of the Functional Independence Measure. *Top Stroke Rehabil* 1994;13:1–15.

20. Wright BD, Linacre JM, Heinemann AW. Measuring functional status in rehabilitation. In: Granger CV, Gresham GE (eds.). *Physical medicine and rehabilitation clinics of North America: new developments in functional assessment.* Philadelphia: Saunders, 1993.

21. Stineman MG, Escarce JJ, Goin JE, Hamilton BB, Granger CV, Williams SK. A case-mix classification system for medical rehabilitation. *Med Care* 1994;32:366–79.

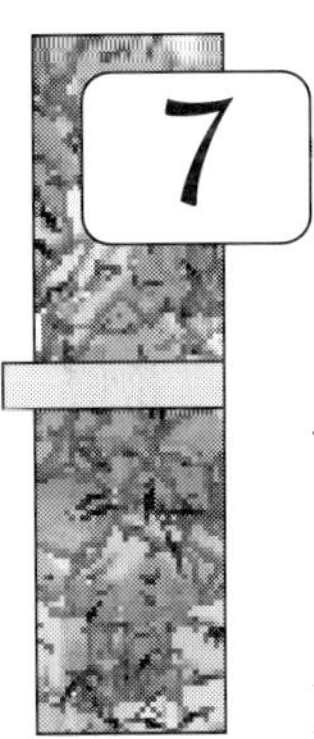

Motor Recovery from Functional Imaging Studies

R. S. J. Frackowiak, M.D.

I will review ideas concerning functional mapping as related to rehabilitation. I am a neurologist who has been interested in the pathophysiology of stroke. Ten years of work has led me to understand that apart from the first three or four hours after ischemia there is little that can be done to salvage tissue as the progression from ischemia to infarction is a rapid process in man.

There is a major opportunity in trying to do something about the disability of stroke and brain injury simply by observing what happens when patients recover, which they all do to a greater or lesser extent. Acute recovery may be ascribed to resolution of edema and reperfusion. What happens during the six months during which slower recovery is occurring? What is happening in the brain that sustains that recovery, and will that give us any clues as to what we should be doing to help rehabilitation?

The first question was how to design an experiment to ask the question, "What is happening in the brain when motor recovery is occurring?" The first confounding problem is that many patients have multiple lesions. The second confounding problem is that even if patients recover well, most will nevertheless perform a task less well than a normal subject. Therefore, a map of what is happening in the brain will be confounded by a performance variable.

The first experiment that we set up explicitly addressed that problem by using patients who recovered completely. Completeness was operationally defined as the ability to perform a finger to thumb opposition task to a given criterion. The criterion was three oppositions per two seconds for two minutes. None of the patients suffered transient ischemic attacks; all had stroke.

We asked a simple question: What happens in the brain when the fingers of the unaffected and recovered hands are moved? We also mapped the finger opposition task in normal subjects and compared this with a map recorded at rest. There is a lateralized system of primary motor cortex, supplementary motor area, a small insular motor area, the basal ganglia activated contralateral to the moving limb and an ipsilateral cerebellar activation. On the other hand, a recovered limb movement results in activity based around the contralateral sensory motor cortex, but the remainder of activity is bilaterally organized. There is activation in bilateral supramarginal gyrus, bilateral insular motor areas, bilateral cerebellum and bilateral premotor areas. This bilaterally organized system also comprises certain areas which are not activated by the same movement with a normal limb.

The next variable that we had to consider was the following: we have a lesion in the brain, we have a functional disability but do we know how the functional disability is subtended by what is going on in the brain? A simple lesion in primary motor cortex or of its outflow is one mechanism, but a lesion in other brain areas causing motor dysfunction may exert its effect by other mechanisms. Does a lesion in the brain just affect the function of that area, or are there distant effects elsewhere in the brain? If there are effects elsewhere, how do they modify the capacity to reorganize? We approached that question, not by using activation methodology, but by using a simple comparison of what is occurring in the brain at rest in patients who have had a lesion, and compared it to the activity in the brain of normal subjects at rest.

We studied a group of patients with lesions of the motor outflow tract in the internal capsule, who had recovered motor function. There was a relative decrease of blood flow compared to the normals in the region of the lesioned internal capsule. In addition to that, there are other areas in the overlying insular motor cortex, the dorsal lateral pre-frontal motor areas, the contralateral cerebellum, in the midbrain and in the brain stem. These are all areas that are functionally and anatomically interconnected and known to be associated with the motor system. Additionally, profound reorganization is occurring in the unlesioned hemisphere, presumably via interhemispheric connections or perhaps via basal ganglia loops.

The issue of disconnections can also be studied with relatively long T2 weighted MRI scans. A twenty-one-year-old patient has been described who had an internal capsule stroke and was profoundly disabled. Over the course of eighteen months he recovered to criterion. He showed degeneration of the pyramidal tract traversing the pons and crossing in the medulla. This man has normal function without a pyramidal tract. He showed on PET scanning the type of redistribution of activity that I have described above. So, when a standard resting blood flow scan is recorded in a patient who has had a stroke, for example in the parietal region, interpretation must be cautious because the resting scan provides limited information. An additional metabolic scan can provide information on the presence or absence of ischemia, pre-ischemia, compensation, etc. Occasionally, phenomena such as cerebellar diaschisis can be seen, but without activation, interpretation is difficult.

We have tried to analyze further what the activation patterns of reorganization essentially mean. Some of the activations may be causative of recovery and others simply associated with the process. Let us consider activation of the ipsilateral motor cortex in recovered patients. This is a group result. If we now go to the individual subjects and we find those subjects who had minor movements in the hand ipsilateral to the infarction during movement of the recovered hand, we find that it is the ones with such involvement that showed bilateral cortical activity. However, bilateral activation in the premotor cortex showed no such association. Clearly, there is a differential implication of these two motor areas in the recovery process.

Can we use data from basic biology to try to interpret why some of the additional areas are activated or not? For example, Goldman Rakic has shown using retrograde labeling of corticospinal pathways in the cortex that there are direct connections to all the areas that I described in the initial activation recovery study, including midline structures, both SMA and cingulate cortices, also in the medial parietal lobe, the supramarginal gyrus, the primary motor cortex, the premotor cortex, and the dorsal lateral prefrontal cortex. So, we can say that those areas activated by the recovered hand movements in addition to the usual areas that are activated with this task have some direct anatomical relationship to the spinal cord. Perhaps they are simply being recruited to perform the task.

Functionally specialized areas of motor associated cortex leave segregated output pathways in the internal capsule. Supplementary motor cortex, primary motor cortex, and premotor cortex fibers can be traced through the internal capsules of monkeys. Supplementary motor cortex fibers pass through the anterior limb of the internal capsule; those from the premotor cortex go through the genu and the anterior third of the posterior internal capsule, and primary motor cortical fibers track through the posterior part of the posterior internal capsule in the monkey. We therefore performed studies on eight new subjects with recovery and looked at the relationship between a lesion site and the pattern of activity that was obtained during movement of the recovered hand. We were able to identify patients with lesions in the posterior half of the posterior end of the internal capsule, and others with a lesion principally in the anterior part or genu of the internal capsule.

There are two essential differences in the associated patterns of cortical activation. Patients with a lesion in the outflow tract from primary motor cortex show an enlargement of the motor output zone that extends into the face area. When the outflow from the primary motor cortex is not lesioned, there is no such enlargement. There is a direct relationship between the anatomy of the lesion and the functional reorganization observed.

We are now beginning to use other diseases to try to understand these structure-function relationships further. We wanted to see whether we could use functional imaging techniques to understand why the motor output zone was enlarged in some patients and not in others. We studied a group of amyotrophic lateral sclerosis patients, because there is degeneration of the pyramidal tract. When they performed similar tasks, we again found an enlargement of the motor output zone in addition to other redistributions of activity. We then carried out a similar experiment with a group of patients with primary muscular atrophy, in which there is degeneration only of the alpha motor neurons and not of the pyramidal tract itself. We matched them in terms of degree of disability to the ALS patients. These patients showed no enlargement of the motor output zone, so that there is enlargement of the motor output zone with posterior internal capsule lesions and complete recovery; enlargement with degeneration of the pyramidal tract and weakness, but no enlargement without degeneration of the pyramidal tract and equivalent weakness. We now have three observations that lead to the conclusion that the enlargement of the motor output zone is due to pyramidal tract damage from primary motor cortex and not to alpha motor neuron loss, impaired proprioceptive feedback, or weakness because they are each controlled in the various observations. This example of the use of lesions and functional imaging in man, in order to try to dissect mechanisms that may be of relevance to the rehabilitation of stroke patients, is illustrative of the use of brain mapping to derive knowledge of potential clinical use.

Let's try to dissect a little further the functions of the other regions that are implicated in the reorganization of cortical function following lesions of the pyramidal tract. There was considerable increase of activity in the supplementary motor area associated with movements of the recovered hand. The supplementary motor area, and indeed the premotor cortex, are very interesting because of their functional association with motor learning. In an experiment that was performed to image the functional anatomy of a movement that is performed naively and then when it becomes automatic through practice, we found the premotor cortex is very interested in the learning phase when it is still performed naively. On the other hand, when that movement becomes automatic, the premotor area is no longer activated, but the supplementary motor area which previously was not active is now massively activated. This observation may be of fundamental importance for how we plan therapies that use feedback learning.

Another region activated when the recovered hand is moved was the dorsal lateral prefrontal cortex. This is a region that is underactive in patients with retarded depression or psychomotor poverty of schizophrenia, i.e., patients who usually do not move unless they are stimulated. There is a decrease in perfusion of this area at rest. The question arises as to whether this area is fundamental to the generation of movements which are not specified by the external environment, but are internally generated, so-called "willed" movements. Subjects placed their hand on the scanning bed in an experiment. During the scanning process, a finger was touched. In one condition, the subject was asked to lift that finger, that is, there was an externally specified response to a sensory stimulus. In the second scan, the patients were instructed "when your finger is touched, move either that finger or the next one, your choice." The movement is the same for both scans, the stimulus is also the same, but the operation in the brain is different. On the one hand, there is an externally driven response, and on the other we have an internally driven response. We recapitulated this formal design in an experiment involving language tasks in order to see whether there was a cross-modal specificity for the willed component of action in the dorsal lateral prefrontal cortex. The result showed activation of dorsal lateral prefrontal cortex in both internally compared to externally driven tasks. There were also specific decreases of activity that were modality specific in the two tasks, with a decrease in primary auditory cortex and the areas behind it in the superior temporal gyrus in the verbal tasks, and in the motor task a deactivation in the primary motor cortex. We appear to show a reciprocally active system involving dorsal lateral prefrontal motor areas and other posterior areas, depending on which task is being performed. Such a result has implications for the way in which therapies are designed, be they internally generated or externally driven tasks.

A final issue that is of importance is how much tissue must be lost before a movement or motor task is no longer performable, given that there is a great redundancy of neural tissue in the brain. This question can be approached in many ways. One way is to make measurements with the subjects performing a motor task at different levels of force. We have scanned subjects with such a paradigm that included six levels of force (10% of maximum, 20%, 30%, 40%, 50%, and 60%). We looked for blood flow changes that correlated with the degree of force exerted during the scans. There are areas in the brain where there is a pronounced correlation of activity with force exerted. These are found in the inferior aspects of the medial premotor and cingulate cortex, in the primary motor cortex itself, in posterior parts of the supplementary motor area, and in the contralateral cerebellum. From such correlations, we can begin to measure the tuning of such motor areas to force or indeed rate or other variables of motor performance.

We can also monitor therapy with functional imaging. An illustration is provided by patients with Parkinson's disease. There are areas of the brain that are not activated when patients perform a particular type of motor task compared to normal subjects. They include the supplementary motor area. We have performed a series of rest and movement tasks while scanning in the presence and absence of a drug that improves motor function. We have shown that as patients obtain benefit from the drug there is activation of the supplementary motor area. Using such combined behavioral, cognitive, and pharmacologic challenges, one can investigate functional/pharmacological interactions directly. Other methods of functional imaging, using dopamine precursor tracers, have allowed monitoring of attempts at modifying function by the introduction of grafted tissue into the brains of Parkinsonian patients.

In summary, functional imaging and informative experimental design in well chosen patient groups is providing novel information of potential use to those interested in recovery of function after brain injury.

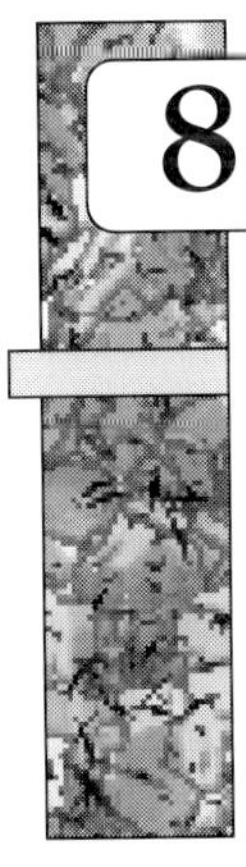

8

The Use of Glucose Metabolic Imaging to Study Central Nervous System Rehabilitation

Amy Garrett and Frank Wood, Ph.D.

Introduction

Functional neuroimaging offers a unique opportunity to advance the understanding of the physiological processes underlying central nervous system rehabilitation. As in all areas of research, however, an understanding of the limitations of the data is essential for proper interpretation. Therefore, scientists who design and analyze imaging studies as well as those who interpret studies conducted in other labs will benefit by being aware of the issues of validity and sources of variance in imaging data. Additionally, some of these issues apply to other methods of research in rehabilitation. In this chapter, we discuss several methodological problems in neuroimaging, and follow with data describing work in progress at our laboratory which addresses these issues.

Validity, both local and global, is the first problem. Locally, we must question the meaning of measuring metabolism at a given level and at a particular site. If measured during task performance, does metabolism indicate the level of competence of the performance? If so, is the correlation positive or negative? Incompetent performance might consume less energy because it simply does not engage the relevant neuronal mechanisms; or, it might generate excess metabolism because inefficient and therefore excessive use is made of the existing neuronal resources. Since both types of relationships have been empirically demonstrated on a variety of tasks, this general question will naturally translate into an empirical one: which behaviors have which relationships to metabolism at which sites? This leads to other important questions of local validity, such as whether a given range of metabolic activation at a given site is necessary or sufficient for accurate task performance.

Questions concerning global validity can be divided into two types: (1) issues about the generalized level of CNS arousal or activation; and (2) issues about the interpretation of relationships between regions, including both positive and negative correlations. In the first case, there is no doubt that some minimal level of metabolic activation is necessary for CNS performance, but it is debatable how to interpret differences in overall activation, either within or between individuals, if those levels are generally

57

within the normal range. The second group of questions introduces the complex and still vague notion of "systems" of interacting regions in the brain. No doubt many neuroanatomical regions participate in producing a given behavior, but the details of that participation remain to be clarified. Obviously, this is especially relevant to rehabilitation, if other regions can "compensate," i.e., support the task performance to a greater degree than would be seen in an undamaged brain.

There is another aspect of validity so complex that it constitutes a separate set of questions. It may be termed the question of summation, both in time and in space. Temporally, an image necessarily accumulates metabolic activity over some time period. As a consequence of that summation, constituent sub-processes of task performance are in principle not identifiable, if their duration is less than that of the period over which the image is summed. Furthermore, almost all neuroimaging paradigms involve repeated execution of some task, and so they necessarily involve periods between the completion of a response and the initiation of the next stimulus-response sequence. This "down time" may nevertheless be filled with all sorts of psychological processes, including expectancy of feedback about correctness of response, anxiety over adequacy of response, and the like. The summed image therefore adds the effect of those processes with the effect of task performance, thereby confounding and complicating the interpretation of the image. Although the extant literature does not abound with demonstrations of the impact of such processes, our own research provides an existence proof of them, thus illustrating their potential importance, at least in some cases. In principle, any functional image sums several constituent sub-processes, only some of which are task-related.

Spatial summation is also an issue in PET, to a far greater extent than in functional MRI because of the superior spatial resolution of function MRI. How best to describe a given region of interest (ROI), particularly if its boundaries are irregular, is still uncertain. What is certain is that partial volume effects are not the only ways in which activity in tissue adjacent to the region of interest may affect measurements in the target region. This problem is greatly affected by the method of back reconstruction of the image: the most common methods substantially blur the image, and allow "bleeding" from adjacent areas into a target area. In the more general case, it remains a question how best to delineate a region of interest, so that the most accurate measurement of the activity within the target boundaries is produced.

Individual differences constitute a third arena of uncertainty about the interpretation of metabolic images relevant to rehabilitation studies. These individual differences include standard competencies of various sorts, on the one hand. These may refer to levels of skill that existed before brain injury; they may also refer to the range of compensatory possibilities possessed by an individual. Individual differences in style or approach to tasks are also highly relevant, including the full range of emotional state and trait variables such as anxiety or depression. Recognition of individual differences typically does not come naturally to neuroscientists, but well over one hundred years of psychological research have demonstrated their strong impact on all areas of life, including education in general and rehabilitation in particular. An additional complication arises when a focal or diffuse brain lesion induces not only primary disabilities in some performance skill but also primary disabilities in emotional self-control, which will usually have a secondary impact on task performance. Disentangling these two sources of task-related incompetency is often a complex problem, no easier to solve when images of metabolic activity are available.

For the past ten years, we have been engaged in a programmatic effort to characterize the neurobehavioral processes involved in dyslexia. This included studies of regional cerebral blood flow profiles in dyslexics and normals, and more recently our research has turned to PET studies of glucose metabolism and functional MRI studies of blood oxygenation. Our experience has brought us to the brink of formal studies of the rehabilitation process in dyslexia, so we have confronted each of the three major types of questions enumerated previously. Accordingly, we venture in this chapter to illustrate some aspects of these problems, insofar as we have encountered them to date or can reasonably anticipate them in the near future.

Task Accuracy Is Related to Regional Activation

Using the xenon inhalation method, we demonstrated that proficiency can be negatively or positively correlated with regional cerebral blood flow (1). In a sample of N = 83 subjects who had been diagnosed as dyslexic in childhood and in N = 69 subjects with no history of reading impairment, better performance of an orthographic (spelling) test administered during 133-xenon inhalation was positively and significantly correlated with left superior temporal cortical blood flow. Childhood reading classification was positively correlated with Wernicke's area activation and negatively correlated with angular gyrus blood flow. Thus, good readers inhibited angular gyrus flow or poor readers excessively activated it, or both. These latter relationships were independent of task accuracy, since only superior temporal flows were related to accuracy. They were not explainable as a marker of improvement in reading since childhood because the relationship held true for both RD subjects who had improved their reading skills and for those whose deficits persisted.

These data can be summarized by showing significant positive correlations between left superior temporal blood flow and phonological/orthographic processes and significant negative correlations between angular gyrus blood flow and comprehension components of reading. Increased ability may be related to increased or decreased regional activation. Another lesson from these data applies specifically to studies of rehabilitation. Subjects who were poor readers in their childhood and then improved by the time of testing showed the same blood flow profile as those who were poor readers in childhood and did not improve. We did not uncover a neurophysiological index of behavioral reading improvement using the 133-xenon inhalation method of measuring cortical blood flow. It is possible that our data analysis missed the rehabilitation-relevant changes. It is also possible that the changes are too subtle to be detected using this method. Certainly, it is preferable to measure physiological change throughout the entire brain. Positron emission tomography (PET) technology offers just that opportunity.

We found another example of the complex relationship between performance and regional physiology using PET imaging studies of glucose metabolism. An adult

Table 8-1. *Positron emission tomography N = 49 normative sample.*

Variable	Minimum	Maximum	Mean	Standard Deviation
Age	20.8	69.0	40.4	13.6
IQ	84.0	136.0	104.6	10.7
Hand	−24.0	24.0	14.2	12.9
Education	10.0	20.0	15.3	2.2
Anxiety	20.0	64.0	30.2	8.3
Task d′	1.8	6.0	3.9	1.1

sample of N = 49 normal volunteers, aged 20-69 years, performed a computerized letter recognition task after [18]-F-2-deoxyglucose (FDG) injection (2). Subjects responded to targets (letters) and refrained from responding to nontarget stimuli (symbols). Table 8-1 provides demographic statistics from this sample.

After the variance associated with the age of the subject was removed, the percentage of hits (correct responses to letters) was significantly and negatively correlated with metabolism in the right inferior temporo-occipital cortex (Area 37) (r = −0.49, p < .006). Thus, the greater percentage of letters correctly identified by a subject, the less he/she activated this visual association area. In contrast, after again accounting for the age of the subject, metabolism in left hemisphere area 37 was significantly and positively related to the percentage of false alarms the subject made during glucose uptake (r = .39, p < .008). The greater the percentage of times that the subject made a mistake by responding to a symbol, the greater the activation of the left hemisphere visual association area.

These data again illustrate that improved performance may be associated with decreased regional metabolism, and also show the importance of considering components of performance (i.e., percentage of hits and false alarms) rather than only a single performance score. Also, it is essential to remove that variance associated with variables such as age to accurately identify behavioral-physiological relationships. This leads us to the next topic of discussion: individual differences analysis.

State and Trait Variables Affect Regional Glucose Metabolism

Data from our lab suggest that both transient affective states and more stable subject traits contribute variance to regional glucose metabolic values (3). By measuring and statistically controlling for the effects of these variables, we gain a more accurate understanding of the interaction between task-related effects and subject variables. Of course, in order to have the statistical power to perform these operations, adequate sample sizes are required. We have the advantage of having collected an exceptionally large database of PET data (N = 49) for the analyses described here.

While dissociation of task-related effects and subject variables such as affective states and personality traits would be ideal, it is difficult to interpret the separate contributions of interacting variables when we sum metabolism over a thirty-five minute window. Therefore, the following data point out the importance of accounting for the effects of individual differences but do not attempt to interpret regional glucose relationships to these variables.

In the experiment described previously, N = 49 normal adult volunteers received PET scans measuring FDG during a letter recognition task. State anxiety was measured just before radiotracer injection using the State Anxiety version of the Speilberger State-Trait Anxiety Inventory (STAI) (4). Each subject also received a neuropsychological test battery and interview. Using the Social Anhedonia Scale of the Chapman and Chapman Schizophrenia Proneness Inventory (5) as well as relevant responses to interview questions, we constructed a score for each subject to measure his or her degree of social withdrawal. Spearman's r correlations were performed using these variables in addition to age, sex, IQ, education, and handedness.

The goal of this analysis was to determine the interrelationships between task variables, subject variables, and regional glucose metabolism. In general, we found that age and state anxiety were related to task performance and to regional metabolic values, while social withdrawal was related to regional values. Furthermore, social withdrawal was related to age.

When we see that individual differences add variance to ROI measurements, analysis of task-related metabolism must be performed by removing this variance. We found that the correlation between percent hits and right Area 37 metabolism is significant only when the variance due to age is removed. The correlation between left Area 37 activation and percent false alarms is increased when age variance is partialled as well.

State anxiety is positively correlated with left hemisphere values of superior dorsolateral prefrontal, area 37, hippocampus, and amygdala, and right orbito-frontal cortex. Before we are tempted to interpret a decrease in right hemisphere or increase in left hemisphere metabolism in state anxiety, we must remove the interacting variance contributed by the percentage of false alarms. Following this, we see that, additionally, right hemisphere hippocampus, amygdala, and dorsolateral prefrontal cortex are also related to anxiety, making interpretation of the data more difficult. Furthermore, the relationship between anxiety and left amygdala metabolism is best described by a polynomial rather than a linear relationship.

Previous studies had shown inverse correlations between anxiety and cerebral blood flow, especially in the frontal right hemisphere (6). An inverted-U relationship between anxiety and frontocortical metabolism (7) and with global CBF (8,9) has been reported, while Giordani et al. (10) reported no effect of anxiety on brain metabolism. We have previously demonstrated the effects of state anxiety on regional blood flow (11). Drevets et al. (12) recently found that anticipatory anxiety increases blood flow in the left striatum, orbital cortex, and thalamus, the right prefrontal cortex, and the bilateral cingulate cortex. Blood flow decreased in the left and right sensorimotor cortex and left insula. These conflicting data suggest that methodological improvements are needed. By measuring and controlling for potential sources of variance, we improve the chances of accurately detecting metabolic correlates of affective states.

Table 8-2. *Sources of variance in glucose metabolic data.*

Variable	Source of Variance	Percent of Variance
Area 37 R	d′	12.6
	age	8.1
Anterior Cingulate L	age	28.3
	social withdrawal	4.5
DorsSupLat L	state anxiety	12.5
	age	8.9
Amygdala L	state anxiety	16.2

Area 37R = right hemisphere Brodmann's Area 37
Anterior Cingulate L = left hemisphere anterior cingulate cortex
DorsSupLatL = left hemisphere superior dorsolateral prefrontal cortex
Amygdala L = left hemisphere amygdaloid complex

Social withdrawal at first glance is seen to be positively correlated with left and right anterior cingulate cortical metabolism and with left hippocampal metabolism. A similar result has been reported previously (13). However, since anterior cingulate metabolism is strongly negatively associated with age (r = −0.51, p < .0001), this confounding variance must be removed before interpretation is possible. After age-related variance is removed, social withdrawal is correlated only with left hippocampal metabolism. We also found that a diagnosis of adult attention deficit disorder (determined by responses to an interview) is negatively correlated with bilateral orbito-frontal metabolism (r =.50, p < .005).

Relationships such as these make it difficult to interpret the separate regional effects of task performance and individual differences. We have shown that age, state anxiety, social withdrawal, and attention deficit disorder affect the glucose metabolic profile and should be measured and accounted for statistically. Table 8-2 lists sources of variance in selected regions of interest. A more thorough analysis of individual difference variability in imaging data is greatly needed.

Individual Differences Are Related to Global Metabolism

The previous discussion showed that individual differences can affect regional glucose metabolism. However, global metabolism is also related to differences between subjects. We have found that both age and a diagnosis of adult ADD are negatively correlated with mean global metabolism (r = −.46, p < .005 for both). Kuhl et al. (14) had previously reported the negative correlation between age and global CBF, while other researchers had found that age does not affect imaging data (15,16). Zametkin (17) previously reported decreased global metabolism in adult ADD subjects, while Lou et al. (18,19) found regional metabolic differences. The effects of global metabolism can be corrected by expressing regional values as percentages of the whole brain mean or by considering global metabolism a covariate in the analysis of regional values. This does not account for differential effects of whole brain metabolism on regional values. It is difficult to interpret the relationship between ADD, for example, and whole brain metabolism. ADD may alter the metabolic profile, resulting in overall lower global values, or may reduce all regional values uniformly. The difficult problem that this presents has no easy solution. At this point, accounting for global mean metabolism by use of regional to whole brain ratios is an essential yet crude statistical control.

Response Components Are Related to Global Metabolism

As discussed previously, the temporal resolution of the PET FDG method is about thirty-five minutes, so a multitude of cognitive processes are recorded in the resulting metabolic profile. One such process may be the subject's psychological reaction to his or her performance. Although this cannot be evaluated neurophysiologically using PET, event-related potentials (ERPs) allow millisecond resolution of brain responses to stimuli. In the normal adult sample described earlier, 16 channel ERPs were recorded while each subject performed the letter recognition task. Therefore, while glucose uptake was measured with PET over thirty-five minutes, ERPs were simultaneously measured in response to each trial and subsequently summed according to the type of stimuli presented (letter or symbol). Components of the ERP were measured and analyzed for relationships to the glucose uptake data.

Among the strongest correlations ($r = .50$, $p < .005$) was that of a negative component peaking at 700 msec post-stimulus (the N700) with global glucose metabolism (20). Since a behavioral response to the stimuli is made around 500 msec, the N700 must be reflecting a post-response process, possibly an evaluative "did I do it right?" response in anticipation of the auditory feedback provided by the computer announcing the correctness of the response. The N700 was relatively high in power (area under the curve squared) compared to other components, which may explain its correlation with global glucose metabolism. More importantly, a cognitive, perhaps evaluative, perhaps anticipatory process not measured behaviorally is affecting the imaging data. Since it is a powerful component of the ERP, it may be contributing significant amounts of variance to the glucose data. This again brings up the question of what cognitive variables are affecting the glucose data. A behavioral or self-report measure of post-response cognitive processes would enable more accurate assessment of the effects of other variables.

The Local Maximum Is a More Accurate Measure of Regional Metabolism Than the Local Average

The resolution of our scanner (about 6 mm) makes it feasible to consider actual anatomical regions of interest rather than slices or boxes within slices. Cerebral activation then connotes a local concentration of active cells within an anatomical region of interest with no implication that the region of interest is activated to the same intensity across its entire domain. Within certain size limits (smaller than

Table 8-3. *Activity measurements for spheres of different sizes.*

Sphere Diameter	Maximum Count	True Maximum	Average Count	True Average	Edge Counte	True Edge*
13 mm	1.9	4.3	2.0	4.3	1.4	2.1
16 mm	2.5	4.3	2.0	4.3	1.8	2.1
22 mm	2.9	4.3	2.3	4.3	1.7	2.1
28 mm	2.6	4.3	2.4	4.3	1.6	2.1
33 mm	3.9	4.3	2.6	4.3	1.8	2.1
38 mm	4.2	4.3	2.9	4.3	1.8	2.1

*The average partial volume for pixels straddling the edge.

a gross anatomical region such as the superior temporal gyrus), the intensity of the activation is considered to be a function of both the number of cells and the activity of those cells. Many scientists define activation as the average of the total voxel values within an anatomical region. Phantom studies conducted in our lab suggest that a more accurate estimate of regional metabolism is the maximum voxel within the ROI (21).

Six spheres ranging in diameter from 13 mm to 38 mm were filled with FDG each with activity of 4.28 microcuries/milliliter. The spheres were immersed in a warm background with activity of 1.03 mcuries/ml. Standard PET images were obtained of the spheres with consecutive image planes of 3.375 mm.

The measurements for each sphere were made from the plane that passed through the center of that sphere. Since the interior diameter of the sphere was known, a circular region of interest was defined that corresponded precisely to the section of the sphere within the plane. Three measurements were made: (1) the average count for all voxels within the sphere; (2) the maximum count within the sphere (the "hottest" voxel); and (3) the average count at the edge of the sphere defined by the voxels that straddled the sphere boundary.

All measurements are presented in Table 8–3. As you can see, for smaller spheres both the calculated average and the measured maximum underestimate the actual activity. The average is a more severe underestimation, however, even though the spheres have the same intensity throughout. The average is low not simply because of a partial volume effect since even voxels safely within the sphere have intensities that are inveresely proportional to their distance from the center of the sphere. Alternatively, the maxima more closely approximate the actual activity even for small spheres and increasingly as the size of the spheres increase. The local maximum may therefore provide a physiologically relevant measure.

We also imaged the Hoffman phantom, which is modeled after a brain and contains regions of uniform "gray matter" with constant intensities that are four times that of the surrounding "white matter." Despite the fact that the larger gray areas were no more intense than the smaller gray areas, they nevertheless were measured as having higher averages and maxima than the smaller gray areas. These data suggest that the local maximum is affected by the size of the ROI. Increased maxima could result from increased activation of a specific area or from a large area of gray matter surrounding the area. We are currently conducting further inquiries to determine the most valid and reliable measure of regional metabolism using the phantom data as well as our N = 49 PET images.

Conclusions

We have reviewed on-going studies from our lab which demonstrate the importance of considering methodological issues in the design, analysis, and interpretation of imaging data. Issues of validity and statistical control of variability are central to any investigation. However they are especially relevant to studies of the neuro-physiological effects of rehabilitation because the changes we seek to detect may be especially complex. An individual rather than a brain structure is the target of rehabilitation, and along with cognitive or motor skills, affective and other psychological processes are affected by both brain injury and rehabilitation. Therefore, although the data discussed above focuses on comparisons between individuals, it is no less valid for studies of changes within an individual. The primary effects of a brain lesion that are most clearly observed through neuropsychological testing interact with the secondary, more subtle effects to produce the behavioral and emotional changes that impair functioning. All of these impairments must be addressed for effective study and treatment.

In summary, we have presented five methodological issues related to rehabilitation imaging research:

1. Task accuracy may be positively or negatively correlated with regional brain activation. Effective task performance requires both sufficient and efficient use of neural resources. Different tasks may increase or decrease metabolism in different structures.

2. Both state and trait variables affect the glucose metabolic profile. Performance, regional metabolism, and individual difference variables interact in producing patterns of activation. All of these variables must be measured and statistically controlled for more accurate interpretation of imaging data.

3. Individual differences affect global metabolism. Both age and a diagnosis of ADD are related to global metabolism. Even though regional metabolism may not be uniformly affected by age and ADD, statistical control of global metabolism is warranted.

4. A subject's psychological response to his or her task performance may add significantly to glucose metabolism variability. Psychological processes that are not behaviorally measured may contribute to and confound imaging data. If two tasks in a subtraction paradigm elicit qualitatively or quantitatively different subjective responses, then the data resulting from the subtraction will be confounded.

5. The local maximum may more closely approximate regional metabolic values than the local average. A consensus on a physiologically valid measure of regional metabolism is needed to standardize measurements of glucose metabolism.

References

1. Flowers DL, Wood FB, Naylor, CE. Regional cerebral blood flow correlates of language processes in reading disability. *Arch Neurol* 1991;48:637–43.
2. Garrett AS, Wood FB, Keyes JW. Glucose metabolism in the inferior temporo-occipital cortex is related to performance on a letter recognition task. Abstract, Society for Neuroscience 25th Annual Meeting, 1995.
3. Garrett AS, Wood FB, Keyes, JW. Anxiety and social inhibition are reflected in regional glucose metabolism as measured by PET. Abstract, Society for Neuroscience 24th Annual Meeting, 1994.
4. Speilberger CD, Gorsuch RL, Luchene R, Bagg PR, Jacobs GA. *Manual for the state-trait anxiety inventory (STAI)—Form Y.* Palo Alto, CA: Consulting Psychologists Press, 1983.
5. Chapman LJ, Chapman JP. Problems in the measurement of cognitive deficit. *Psych Bull* 1973;79:380-85.
6. Rodriguez G, Cogorno P, Gris A, et al. Regional cerebral blood flow and anxiety: a correlation study in neurologically normal patients. *J Cereb Blood Flow Metab* 1989;9:410-16.
7. Reivich M, Gur R, Alavi A. Positron tomographic studies of sensory stimuli, cognitive processes and anxiety. *Human Neurobiology* 1983;2:25–33.
8. Gur RC, Gur RE, Resnick SM, Skolnick BE, Alavi A, Reivich M. The effect of anxiety on cortical cerebral blood flow and metabolism. *J Cereb Blood Flow Metab* 1987;7(2):173–77.
9. Gur RC, Gur RE, et al. Effects of task difficulty on regional cerebral blood flow: relationships with anxiety and performance. *Psychophysiology* 1988;25(4):392–99.
10. Giordani B, Boivin MJ, et al. (1990) Anxiety and cerebral cortical metabolism in normal persons. *Psychiatry Research: Neuroimaging* 1990;35:49–60.
11. Wood FB, Flowers DL. Hypofrontal vs. hypo-sylvian blood flow in schizophrenia. *Schizophrenia Bulletin* 1990;16(3):413–24.
12. Drevets WC, Videen TO, Snyder AZ, MacLeod AK, Raichle ME. Regional cerebral blood flow changes during anticipatory anxiety. Abstract, Society for Neuroscience 24th Annual Meeting, 1994.
13. Gottschalk LA, Fronczek J, Abel L, Buchsbaum MS. The relationship between social alienation and disorganized thinking in normal subjects and localized cerebral glucose metabolic rates assessed by positron emission tomography. *Comprehensive Psychiatry* 1992;33(5):332–41.
14. Kuhl DE, Metter EJ, Riege WH, Phelps MS. Effects of human aging on patterns of local cerebral glucose utilization determined by the [18–F] fluorodeoxyglucose method. *J Cereb Blood Flow Metab* 1982;2:163–71.
15. Hatazawa J, Brooks RA, Di Chiro G, Campbell G. Global cerebral glucose utilization is independent of brain size: a PET study. *J Computer Assisted Technology* 1987;11(4):571-76.
16. Duara F, Gross-Glenn K, Barker W, Loewenstein D, Chang J. PET studies during reading in dyslexics and controls. *Neurology* 39 (Supp 1):165.
17. Zametkin AJ, Nordahl TE, Gross M, King AC, Semple WE, Rumsey J, Hamburger S, Cohen RM. Cerebral glucose metabolism in adults with hyperactivity of childhood onset. *New Engl J Med* 1990;323(20):1361–1415.
18. Lou HC, Henriksen L, Bruhn P. Focal cerebral hypoperfusion in children with dysphasia and/or attention deficit disorder. *Arch Neurol* 1984;41:825–29.
19. Lou HC, Henriksen L, Bruhn P, Borner H, Nielsen JB. Striatal dysfunction in attention deficit and hyperkinetic disorder. *Arch Neurol* 1989;46:48–52.
20. Wood FB, Garrett AS, Hart LA, Flowers DL, Absher JR. Event-related potential correlates of glucose metabolism in normal adults during a cognitive activation task. In press. 1995.

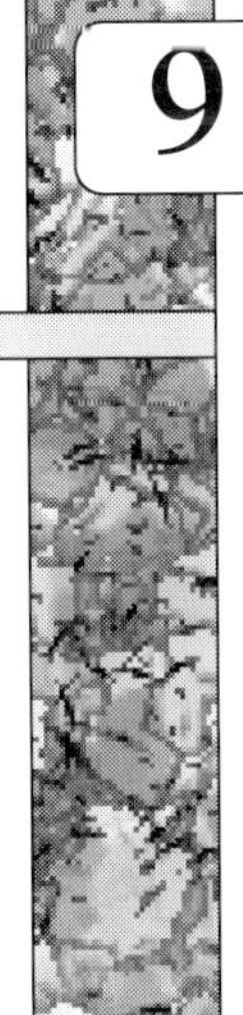

9

The Potential of Combining Diffusion and T_2 Magnetic Resonance Imaging to Satisfy the Requirements of Acute Stroke Assessment: An Analysis

K. M. A. Welch, M.D.

Introduction

Magnetic resonance (MR) technology is now highly advanced in imaging brain structure and progress has been made in the imaging of function. Recently developed MR techniques may be of use not only to diagnose stroke, but also in the assessment of stroke prior to innovative treatments such as with thrombolytic and cytoprotective drugs. The clinician who treats acute stroke requires an imaging technique for the rapid and early identification of stroke. If the same imaging technique were to provide an early and reliable prediction of eventual ischemic cell damage and volume of infarction, it would be of immense value for judging the effectiveness of therapy. Cerebral blood flow (CBF), CT scanning, and metabolic imaging have limited clinical acceptability in this regard. Along the same lines but with a different approach, some clear marker of the state and extent of tissue viability remaining would be valuable to judge if therapy may still be worthwhile when patients are studied at later times after stroke onset. Time alone is an inadequate indicator of the therapeutic window, especially when the time of stroke onset is uncertain. Thus, there is a need to *predict the evolution* of stroke in a way that more precisely and with greater resolution identifies the progression of cellular damage at the moment of investigation. This also would be of value for treatments such as thrombolysis when knowledge of the degree and extent of tissue necrosis and the consequent potential for brain hemorrhage is of utmost importance.

For the acute management of stroke it is desirable to have one measuring device, thereby shortening the time of the early investigative process and permitting treatment at the earliest possible time. This device should be readily available, rapid, and non invasive, and should provide the maximum number of measurements, including diagnostics. High field magnets ($\geq$ 1.5 Tesla) are now installed in general hospitals throughout the world. Magnetic resonance technology at these field strengths can observe anatomical structure, identify arterial occlusion, and measure CBF, metabolism, and integrity of the blood–brain barrier. Currently, however, the technology is such that it would occupy hours of study to achieve this complete information in one session. The challenge is to reduce (1) the time of the MR methods, or (2) identify the most critically important measures for the diagnosis, staging, and prediction of outcome of stroke, or both.

Existing Techniques

It is pertinent to briefly review and critique those procedures that may be already available and tested for their potential to provide an early prediction of eventual tissue infarction after onset of ischemia. CT scanning is limited because it is unable to detect the ischemic focus acutely. CBF measurement, although predictive of neurologic deficit at the onset of ischemia (1), and despite the strong associations found between the degree and duration of CBF reduction and irreversible cell death in rigorously controlled and reproducible stroke models (2), has limited utility in clinical patients. This is due not only to the time delay between stroke onset and the time of study or to the heterogeneity of CBF in human ischemic foci caused by such factors as variable collateral vasocapacitance and reperfusion, but also the initial ischemic insult activates a cascade of cellular events that apparently proceed independent of the subsequent CBF levels (3). Measures of CBF combined with blood volume and brain oxygen consumption using PET provide information on regions of "misery perfusion" in which the fraction of the O_2 extraction is indicative of cell viability (4). But PET scanners are not in general clinical use and the measurements are often time-consuming. Further, PET cannot provide routine diagnostic measures, unlike MR, and employs radioactive tracers. Metabolic imaging is not developed for MR systems but, due to low signal-to-noise, these measurements have limited resolution, particularly in the case of 31-Phosphorus spectroscopic imaging. Study times are also lengthy. The NAA measured by ^1H MR spectroscopy has been proposed as a marker of cell death (5) but accordingly should be more useful in measuring outcome of ischemia rather than predicting outcome. Thus there is a need to search for new approaches to predict stroke that will have greater clinical application in the acutely ill patient.

Magnetic Resonance of Ischemia

Magnetic resonance can noninvasively measure specific parameters that are sensitive to the biophysical environment of water in tissue (6). These include the water ^1H spin-lattice (T_1) and spin-spin (T_2) relaxation times, spin density (SD), and the translational (apparent) diffusion coefficient (ADC_W) . Magnetic resonance imaging (MRI) readily identifies change in the ^1H NMR parameters of water which occur following ischemic stroke (7-18). There is a progressive increase in T_2 which, however, does not maximize until approximately twenty-four hours after onset. Similar results have been found for changes in T_1; proton spin density increases are observed even later (9).

The acute increase in T$_2$ following ischemia forms the basis for the diagnostic utility of MRI in ischemic stroke. This is thought to be caused by developing vasogenic edema, but the mechanisms remain to be determined. Unlike the increase in T$_1$ relaxation time, which reflects the accumulation of bulk water, T$_2$ changes are influenced by protein content of the fluid as ischemia evolves. Also, using the methodology of ^{1}H magnetization transfer contrast (MTC) imaging (19), our laboratory has shown that decrease in bound intracellular water may be a contributing factor, possibly because of ischemic changes in the cellular environment, e.g., protein breakdown. Whatever the mechanisms, the clinical diagnosis of stroke uses techniques that generate T$_2$-weighted images, considered the "gold standard" measure because of the conformity of T$_2$-weighted MR images with histopathological identification of ischemic lesions postmortem (20,21).

Recently MRI has been adapted to generate images whose contrast is based on the translational motion (diffusion) of water and, thus, may be more specific for tissue characterization (22). Diffusion is a process whereby water molecules move in a random fashion due to thermal energy (Brownian motion). Intra Voxel Incoherent Motion (IVIM), based on the Pulsed Gradient Spin Echo (PGSE) technique developed originally by Stejskal and Tanner (23), has been developed to generate images that can be used to calculate the apparent diffusion coefficient of water (ADC$_W$). In brain, the diffusion of water is impeded by cellular membranes, organelles, macromolecules, and other cellular structures. The intensity of diffusion images thus depends on such factors as tortuosity of the diffusion path, cell membrane permeability, and the exchange of free with bound water.

The diffusion imaging technique has been used to study cerebral ischemia (7–12), which, shortly after onset, causes a decline in the ADC$_W$ by approximately a factor or two, representing a *decrease* in the translational movement of water. This decline is rapid (within minutes) and precedes changes in any other ^{1}H NMR parameters. Moseley et al. (7) reported that the ADC$_W$ declines significantly within the first three minutes after middle cerebral artery occlusion (MCA-O) in the cat, and that by twelve minutes after ischemia the ADC$_W$ falls by 25–30%. Additionally, Mintorovitch et al. (24) demonstrated that acute decreases in the ADC$_W$ were independent of changes in total brain water content, although increases in brain water content occurred after sixty minutes of MCA-O occlusion. Thus ADC$_W$ measurements are sensitive to changes in the environment of water independent of changes in total water content. Our studies have shown that during severe permanent focal ischemia in the rat, after an initial fall the ADC$_W$ values begin to recover toward the normal range after the elapse of eight to twenty-four hours and then attain values that are higher than normal over seven days. Similar changes, although with a much protracted time course, have been recorded in human stroke (25) (see later discussion).

There is considerable interest in the mechanism(s) responsible for the ischemia-induced decline in ADC$_W$, but the physical basis for these changes remains to be determined. A full discussion of these mechanisms is beyond the scope of this chapter, but, in brief, proposed mechanisms include temperature effects, increased tortuosity of the extracellular diffusion paths, restriction by reduced cellular membrane permeability, shifts in water from extracellular to intracellular space, membrane depolarization and cytotoxic edema (11,12,26–38). The rapidity of the decline in the ADC_W after ischemia suggests that, at least initially, it is not a result of the gross secondary changes in ischemic tissue histopathology such as vasogenic edema or tissue necrosis.

The decline in the ADC_W following cerebral ischemia is associated with a specific threshold level of rCBF. Using bilateral common carotid artery occlusion in the gerbil (11), it was demonstrated that the decline in the ADC_W did not begin until rCBF (measured by H_2-clearance) had reached a level of approximately 15 mg/100⁻¹ per minute, a threshold similar to that which is associated with the loss of membrane potential. Increased signal intensity of DWI was also associated with breakdown of energy metabolism, acidosis, cellular ionic shifts, and decreased Na^+, K^+, ATPase activity (39). Such ionic and metabolic changes at critical CBF thresholds have been well established previously using techniques other than MR (1) and are coincident with the onset of neurological deficit. Thus, ADC_W decrease is closely associated with CBF decrease and metabolic impairment in the early minutes and possibly early hours of ischemia. The association between ADC_W, CBF, and cerebral metabolism as ischemia progresses, as well as relationships of each alone or in combination, to histopathologic damage remain to be determined.

The mechanism(s) responsible for the rise is ADC_W subsequent to the initial decrease have been less intensively studied but logically may be a reversal of those responsible for its initial decline as well as impairment of those processes responsible for the physiological restriction of brain water diffusion. The ADC_W increase may mark the disruption of cell membrane structure, necrosis, and loss of cells (i.e., the breakdown of barriers to diffusion) and will be discussed later.

There have been few published studies of DWI in human stroke. Chien et al. (40) investigated fifteen patients with focal cerebral ischemia and infarction within twenty-four hours [n = 3] and up to four years, some studied serially [n = 4]. They found an increase of the "average ADC_W" in ischemic lesions compared to normal controls at these subacute and chronic times of study, observing further increases as time progressed. They attributed this to vasogenic edema complicating the subacute strokes and to gliosis or encephalomalacia in the two- to four-year-old strokes. On the other hand, Warach et al. (25) studied thirty-two ischemic stroke patients with different techniques, at times from two to twelve hours [n = 12] and up to twelve days, in whom the ADC_W ratio, calculated as the ADC_W in homologous brain regions divided by that of the stroke region, was low acutely, reached a nadir at twenty-four hours, and then remained low. There was then no change in ADC_W up to two months but chronic infarcts had a relative increase in ADC_W, although not until four months. The differences in these results can probably be explained on technical grounds, as well as by the use of different controls. Indeed, the control values of Warach et al. (25) were higher than expected, although the use of ratios adjusted for this in part. Both studies had small numbers of patients, particularly at the early time points of the investigation. The techniques used were less advanced than those currently available so that, for example, movement artifact could not be easily corrected and only two images were available for calculation of the ADC_W. Further, measuring an average ADC_W value from a single locus of an ischemic focus of well-known heterogeneity may add to the variability. Nevertheless, although the interpretation of their findings is limited by the aforementioned problems, these were seminal studies in the application of DWI to human stroke.

Our own studies are more in accord with those of Chien et al. (40). In the majority of our patients, we observed an increase of ADC_W as early as twenty-four hours after stroke onset, but a prolonged decrease of ADC_W was found in one-third. Similar findings have been reported in abstract form by the Moseley group (41). Thus, although more extensive investigations are required in clinical patients at all stages of stroke evolution, it appears that the average ADC_W in human ischemic foci may be decreased at acute times of investigation, subsequently to rebound to increased levels as ischemia evolves to cellular necrosis. Although the directions of ADC_W change are the same as in animal models of ischemia, it remains to be determined if the degree and duration of change is the same and to what extent heterogeneity of ADC_W change is present in an ischemic focus. The ADC_W findings in clinical patients will now be discussed, together with the findings in experimental animal models for their potential to characterize and predict ischemic tissue damage.

MR Correlates of Ischemic Histopathology

There is evidence that DWI and quantification of ADC_W may predict histopathological outcome of cerebral ischemia (9,27,42–47). Sevick et al. (46) showed that DWI signal intensity correlated with lack of lesion staining by 2,3,5-triphenyltetrazolium chloride (TTC). Minematsu et al. (47) showed similar findings in the rat MCA-O model. Conventional NMR using T_2 obtained during the stage of cerebral infarction correlates well with the histopathology of the lesion (20,21). This is despite the fact that T_2 essentially characterizes vasogenic edema rather than cellular change, so that it is insensitive to ischemic tissue damage before vasogenic edema develops. Further, the stroke region appears homogeneous on T_2WI and it is usually impossible to detect different regions of tissue damage in the lesion. On the other hand, ADC_W is sensitive to early ischemia and can reveal heterogeneity in regions of ischemia that are homogeneous on T_2WI (42). ADC_W alone can provide earlier and more specific information on regional ishemic histopathology, particularly when shifts in values can be observed over time (50).

Our laboratory has expended a major experimental effort to examine the relationships of MR measures to tissue histopathology in rat models of permanent and transient focal cerebral ischemia (9,19,27,43,44,48–50). We are one of few laboratories to have successfully accomplished serial measures over prolonged time periods of up to one week. These studies have provided strong support that DWI may be a powerful tool in predicting ischemic histopathology. The data obtained in these experiments indicated a reduction in ADC_W, with gradation of change in terms of time and degree from minimally to severely injured tissue. Elevation of T_2 seemed to follow a similar gradation of change that was delayed compared to ADC_W. It is especially interesting to note that in the most heavily injured areas the value of ADC_W began to turn toward normal values, coincident with the emergence of eosinophilic neurons which signify neuronal damage. The subsequent increase of ADC_W, therefore, probably indicates a loss of cell membrane integrity (i.e., allowing the unrestricted movement of water molecules) and cell necrosis. According to our results, the ability to distinguish the return toward normal ADC_W caused by injury from the return of ADC_W to normal that is expected of recovery is dependent on T_2 changes which, when elevated, represent the former. A major point to be made is that high ADC_W and high T_2 together represent cellular necrosis. Even when T_2 subsequently declines toward normal values, the ADC_W remains elevated and remains a signature of cellular necrosis. In this instance what causes T_2 decline from previously elevated values in severely damaged tissue remains to be determined, but possibly reflects decrease of vasogenic edema or a shortening of T_2 relaxation properties because of paramagnetic elements in the tissues such as red blood cells from the petechial hemorrhage associated with tissue necrosis.

Further studies in the rat model of MCA-O have shown that after permanent occlusion for two hours (44), a low ADC_W predicts to a high degree of probability cellular necrosis at one week measured histopathologically. However, a low ADC_W at one hour was not predictive. This study taken together with the results obtained above offers important conclusions for the interpretation of human stroke data.

1. A low ADC_W in acute stroke can be associated with the potential for cellular recovery, eventual cell necrosis, or both, dependent on subsequent ischemic events, and thus, if used alone, has a low probability of predicting cell necrosis.
2. A low ADC_W with high T_2 as ischemia progresses may have a better probability of predicting, but is not a marker for, eventual cell necrosis, although events leading to irreversible cell death may or may not have commenced.
3. High ADC_W and high T_2 is a marker of cell necrosis in the tissue and the time between the transition from low to high ADC_W values probably marks the onset and progression of cell necrosis, although irreversible cell death may have occurred prior to this time.

Clinical Application

In clinical practice, stroke patients cannot be studied at the precise time of stroke onset or serially over prolonged time periods so that moment to moment shifts in ADC_W cannot be observed. Instead a "snapshot" of events is obtained at the earliest possible time and possibly on one or two other occasions during a stroke evaluation. Thus, based on experimental observations (50), at these less acute time points the ADC_W in tissue destined for necrosis may be low, normal, or high as the ADC_W shifts from low to high values, and there will be a heterogeneous distribution of ADC_W values throughout central and peripheral regions. Further, there must be some measure to discriminate a "normal" value of ADC_W in its transition to high values in regions undergoing active cellular necrosis from that of normal ADC_W values in recovering tissue. For these reasons another complementary measure, perhaps more than one, is likely to be important to characterize the evolving ischemic histopathology. We believe that the combined measurement of ADC_W with T_2 will achieve these aims. The biophysical mechanisms of T_2 change are better known than those of the ADC_W (6). The

T correlates of histopathology, although regionally and dynamically limited, are established (20,21).

At the outset it is important to note that there are different time courses of change between ADC$_W$ and T$_2$ (50), which provide support that the ADC$_W$ is influenced by factors other than bulk flow of water. So it is possible to observe low ADC$_W$ in the presence of T$_2$, indicating that ADC$_W$ remains sensitive to cellular change when T$_2$ is influenced by vasogenic edema. In the early stages of cerebral ischemia, before the development of vasogenic edema, ADC$_W$ is decreased without change in T$_2$ (50). Although a low ADC$_W$ has been associated with some form of cellular change, it is uncertain what level of damage is needed to bring about ADC$_W$ reduction. Data from reperfusion models of focal cerebral ischemia suggest that low ADC$_W$ is sensitive not only to eventual cell death, but also to a degree of cellular impairment that is compatible with cell recovery (44). The predictive probability of ADC$_W$ is also influenced by the degree and time course of ADC$_W$ reduction, as well as the region of the lesion (44,50). In acute human stroke, studied before vasogenic edema develops, i.e., before T$_2$ elevation, the potential for cellular recovery in regions of low ADC$_W$ would be supported if the volume of the eventual infarct were less than the volume of early ADC$_W$ reduction. It should also be possible to identify the regionality of recovery probability, perhaps present in more peripheral zones. On the one hand, the knowledge that a low ADC$_W$ does not rule out the potential for cell recovery is encouraging for the use of ADC$_W$ to monitor the effects of cytoprotective drugs. On the other hand, however, the documentation that a low ADC$_W$ can be caused by a spectrum of cellular change from potentially reversible metabolic deficit to destined cell necrosis (45) means that in clinical practice other measures may be essential to discriminate degrees of recoverability, especially at later times of study.

Experimental studies have shown, now confirmed by human stroke observations, that as ischemia progresses and T$_2$ becomes elevated, ADC$_W$ may remain low (50). Whether the development of vasogenic edema and consequent increase of T$_2$ in the presence of a low ADC$_W$ predicts that the tissue has undergone irreversible ischemic damage remains to be determined. Van Bruggen et al. (42) studied a photoactivation model of focal cerebral infarction and found that a hyperintense rim of the lesion seen on DWI was associated with edema without cell necrosis. Pierpaoli et al. (45) found, to the contrary in the same model, that this region was associated with cell necrosis identified by electronmicroscopy. The latter investigation also showed that the same MR characteristics were present in the necrotic core of the lesion in the earlier time course of its evolution. We have shown in a more representative model of focal ischemia that (27,50) in core regions of the lesion, low ADC$_W$ in the presence of high T$_2$ is a predictor of eventual ischemic necrosis. But in the peripheral zones of the lesion, an initial reduction of ADC$_W$ occurred in tissue that had minor histopathological change, but in which T$_2$ was minimally or not increased after ADC$_W$ had recovered.

Thus, it remains to be determined whether a low ADC$_W$ and high T$_2$ has histopathological correlates in human stroke of (1) vasogenic edema in ischemic regions destined from recovery, (2) eventual cell necrosis, or (3) both (dependent on stroke region). We *postulate that this signature represents a probable predictor of cell necrosis.* Were this known, it would have important implications for human stroke assessment. First, when brain regions are identified with this signature, although the cascade of events leading to cell necrosis may have begun, there may still be some potential benefit from cytoprotective drugs working at later points in the cascade, perhaps in more peripheral zones of the ischemic focus. Secondly, cellular necrosis has not yet occurred in these brain regions so perhaps there will be less compliance of these tissues to hemorrhagic conversion or massive enhancement of vasogenic edema after reperfusion therapy. These hypotheses can all be investigated in clinical stroke using the combined measures ADC_W/T_2 and the ability of ADC_W to discriminate cellular ischemic change in the presence of vasogenic edema.

At some time in the course of permanent ischemia, which appears to depend on the duration and degree of ischemia as well as the region of the lesion forming in the distribution of the occluded artery, the ADC_W value begins to return toward the normal range and then becomes abnormally high due to cell loss and tissue necrosis (50). Our animal data strongly supports that this "flip-flop" of ADC_W from low to high values is associated with necrosis of cells in which it occurs. Therefore, if a snapshot image is taken in later stages of clinical stroke evolution when cellular necrosis has occurred, we can expect to find regions of high T_2 in association with ADC_W values in a normal range, in which tissue the ADC_W had been low previously. This will be a marker of active cell necrosis and also of the transition to established necrosis, which is characterized by a high ADC_W in association with a high T_2.

Conclusions

The significance of an available predictor and marker of cell necrosis cannot be overemphasized. T_2WI has been unable to discriminate regions of necrosis from less involved tissue in a subacute ischemic focus, which is essential if MR is to be used for other than diagnostic purposes in stroke patients. In combination with DWI, however, it opens the possibility to identify tissue that may respond to cytoprotective therapy, and perhaps extend the therapeutic window or open it for those cases in whom the time of stroke onset cannot be determined with certainty. At the least, such tissue signatures might indicate, at subacute stages of stroke, whether the total lesion is beyond recovery. This review indicates that DWI together with T_2WI can identify both reversible and irreversible components of the ischemic lesion, in which the response of the reversible component to cytoprotective therapy can be revealed and monitored by the same MR measures.

References

1. Astrup J, Siesjö BK, Symon L. Thresholds in cerebral ischemia—the ischemic penumbra. *Stroke* 1981;12:723.
2. Marcoux FW, Morawetz RB, Crowell RM, DeGirolami U, Halsey JH. Differential regional vulnerability in transient focal cerebral ischemia. *Stroke* 1982;13:339–46.
3. Welch KMA, Barkley GL. Biochemistry and pharmacology of cerebral ischemia. In: Barnett HJM, Mohr JP, Stein MB, Yatsu FM (eds.). *Stroke: pathophysiology, diagnosis, and management*. New York: Churchill Livingstone, 1986:75–90.

4. Baron JC, Frackowiak RSJ, Herholz K, Jones T, Lammertsma AA, Mazoyer B, Wienhard K. Use of PET methods for measurement of cerebral energy metabolism and hemodynamics in cerebrovascular disease. *J Cereb Blood Flow Metab* 1989;9:723–42.

5. Nadler JV, Cooper JR. N-Acetyl-aspartic acid content of human neural tumours and bovine peripheral nervous tissue. *J Neurochem* 1972;19:313–19.

6. Mansfield P, Morris PG. Water in biological systems. In: Waugh JS (ed.). *NMR imaging in biomedicine*. London: Academic Press, 1982:15–31.

7. Moseley ME, Cohen Y, Mintorovitch J, Chileuitt L, Shimizu H, Mucharczyk J, Wendland MF, Weinstein PR. Early detection of regional cerebral ischemia in cats: comparison of diffusion- and T_2-weighted MRI and spectroscopy. *Mag Reson Med* 1990;14:330-46.

8. Shimizu H, Chileuitt L, Mintorovitch J, Cohen J, Moseley ME, Weinstein PR. Early detection of cerebral ischemia by diffusion-weighted MRI after middle cerebral artery occlusion and reperfusion in rats. *J Neurosurg* 1990;72:36A.

9. Knight RA, Ordidge RJ, Helpern JA, Chopp M, Rodolosi LC, Peck D. Temporal evolution of ischemic damage in rat brain measured by proton magnetic resonance imaging. *Stroke* 1991;22:802–808.

10. Moseley ME, Mintorovitch J, Asgari H, Vexler Z, Kucharczyk J. Diffusion/perfusion MR characterization of hyperacute cerebral ischemia. *Proceedings of the Xth annual meeeting of the Soc of Magn Reson Med* 1991;1:330.

11. Busza AL, Allen KL, Gadian DG, Crockard HA. Early changes demonstrated by diffusion-weighted MR imaging in experimental cerebral ischemia. *Proceedings of the Xth annual meeting of the Soc of Magn Reson Med* 1991;1:328.

12. Benveniste H, Hedlund IW, Johnson GA. Mechanism of detection of acute cerebral ischemia in rats by diffusion-weighted magnetic resonance microscopy. *Stroke* 1992;23:754–56.

13. Naruse S, Horikawa Y, Tanaka C, Hirakawa K, Hiroyasu N, Yoshizaki K. Proton nuclear magnetic resonance studies of brain edema. *J Neurosurg* 1982;56:747–52.

14. Buonanno FS, Pykett IL, Brady TJ, Vielma J, Burt CT, Godman MR, Hinsaw WS, Pohost GM, Kisler JP. Proton NMR imaging in experimental ischemic infarction. *Stroke* 1983;14.178–94.

15. Mano I, Levy RM, Crooks LE, Hosobuichi Y. Proton nuclear magnetic resonance imaging of acute experimental cerebral ischemia. *Invest Radiol* 1983;17:345–51.

16. Horikawa Y, Naruse S, Tanaka C, Hirakawa K, Hiroyasu N. Proton NMR relaxation times in ischemic brain edema. *Stroke* 1986;17:1149–52.

17. Bederson JB, Bartkowski HM, Meen K, Halks-Miller M, Nishimura MC, Brant-Zawadski M, Pitts LH. Nuclear magnetic resonance imaging and spectroscopy in experimental brain edema in a rat model. *J Neurosurg* 1986;64:795–801.

18. Kato H, Kogure K, Ohtomo H, Izumiyama M, Tobita M, Matsui S, Yamamoto E, Kohno H, Idebe Y, Wantanabe T. Characterization of experimental ischemic brain edema utilizing proton nuclear magnetic resonance imaging. *J Cereb Blood Flow Metab* 1986;6:212–21.

19. Ordidge RJ, Helpern JA, Knight RA, Qing Z, Welch KMA. Investigation of cerebral ischemia using magnetization transfer contrast (MTC) MR imaging. *Magn Reson Imag* 1991;9:895–902.

20. Bose B, Jones SC, Lorig R, Friel HT, Weinstein M, Little JR. Evolving focal cerebral ischemia in cats: spatial correlation of nuclear magnetic resonance imaging, cerebral blood flow, tetrazolium staining, and histopathology. *Stroke* 1988;19:28–37.

21. Brant-Zawadzki M, Pereira B, Weinstein P, et al. MR imaging of acute experimental ischemia in cats. *AJNR* 1986;7:7–11

22. LeBihan D, Breton E, Lallemand D, Grenier P, Cabanis E, Laval-Jeantet M. MR imaging of intravoxel incoherent motions: application to diffusion and perfusion in neurologic disorders. *Radiology* 1986;161:401–407.

23. Stejskal EO, Tanner JE. Spin diffusion measurements: spin-echoes in the presence of a time dependent field gradient. *J Phys Chem* 1965;42:288–92.

24. Mintorovitch J, Baker LL, Yang GY, Shimizu H, Weinstein PR, Moseley ME, Kucharczyk J. Diffusion-weighted hyperintensity of early cerebral ischemia: correlation with brain water content and ATPase activity. *Proc Soc Magn Reson Med* 1991;10:329 (abstract).

25. Warach S, Chien D, Li W, Ronthal M, Edelman RR. Fast magnetic resonance diffusion-weighted imaging of acute human stroke. *Neurology* 1992;42:1717–23.

26. Moonen CT, Pekar J, de Vleeschouwer MH, van Gelderen P, van Zijl PC, DesPres D. Restricted and anisotropic displacement of water in healthy cat brain and in stroke studied by NMR diffusion imaging. *Magn Reson Med* 1991;19:327–32.

27. Helpern JA, Dereski MO, Knight RA, Ordidge RJ, Chopp M, Qing MS. Histological correlations of nuclear magnetic resonance imaging parameters in experimental cerebral ischemia. *Magn Reson Imag* 1993;11:241–46.

28. Lynch LJ. Water relaxation in heterogeneous and biological systems. In: Cohen JS (ed.). *Magnetic resonance in biology*, Volume 2. New York: John Wiley:280–96.

29. Kuntz ID, Kauzmann W. Hydration of proteins and polypeptides. In: Anfinsen CB, Edsall JR, Richards FM (eds.). *Advances in protein chemistry*, Volume 28. New York: Academic Press:314–15.

30. Inuzuka T, Tamura A, Sato S, Kirino T, Yanagisawa K, Toyoshima I, Miyatake T. Changes in the concentrations of cerebral proteins following occlusion of the middle cerebral artery in rats. *Stroke* 1990;21:917–22.

31. Fung LWM, Narasimhan C, Lu HZ, Weaterman MP. Reduced water exchange in sickle cell anemia red cells: a membrane abnormality. *Biochem Biophys Acta* 1989;982:167–72.

32. Benga G, Morariu VV. Membrane defect affecting water permeability in human epilepsy. *Nature* 1977;265:636–38.

33. Serbu AM, Marian A, Popescu O, Pop VI, Borza V, Benga I, Benga GH. Decreased water permeability of erythrocyte membranes in patients with Duchenne muscular dystrophy. *Muscle & Nerve* 1986;9:127.

34. Fritz OG Jr, Swift TJ. The state of water in polarized and depolarized nerves. *Biophys J;* 7:675–87.

35. Tanner JE. Transient diffusion is a system partitioned by permeable barriers. Application to NMR measurements with a pulsed field gradient. *J Chem Phys* 1978;69(4):1748–54.

36. Tanner JE, Stejskal EO. Restricted self-diffusion of protons in colloidal systems by the pulsed-gradient, spin-echo method. *J Chem Phys*;49(4):1768–77.

38. Tanner JE. Self-diffusion of water in grog muscle. *Biophys J* 1979;28:107–16.

39. Moseley ME, Brant-Zawadzki M, Berry I, Bartkowski H, Weinstein P, Germano I, Nishimura MC, Chew W, Hurd R, Levy R. Magnetic resonance imaging and 31-P and 1-H spectroscopy of experimental brain ischemia. *Am J Neuroradiol* 1986;7:538–39.

40. Chien D, Kwong KK, Gress DR, Buonanno FS, Buxton RB, Rosen BR. MR diffusion imaging of cerebral infarction in humans. *AJNR* 1992;13:1097–1102.

41. de Crespigny A, Yenari M, Enzmann D, Marks S, Moseley M. Navigated spin-echo diffusion imaging of human stroke. *SMRM*, Abstract 1347, 1994.

42. van Bruggen N, Cullen BM, King MD, Doran M, Williams SR, Gadian DG, Cremer JE. T_2- and diffusion-weighted magnetic resonance imaging of a focal ischemic lesion in rat brain. *Stroke* 1992;23:576–82.

43. Dereski MO, Chopp M, Knight RA, Rodolosi LC, Garcia JH. The heterogeneous temporal evolution of focal ischemic neuronal damage in the rat. *Acta Neuropathol* 1993;85:327–33.

44. Jiang Q, Zhang ZG, Chopp M, Helpern JA, Ordidge RJ, Garcia JH, Marchese BA, Qing ZX, Knight RA. Temporal evolution and spatial distribution of the diffusion constant of water in rat brain after transient middle cerebral artery occlusion. *J Neurol Sci* 1993;120:123–30.
45. Pierpaoli C, Righini A, Linfante I, Tao-Cheng JH, Alger JR, Di Chiro G. Histopathologic correlates of abnormal water diffusion in cerebral ischemia: diffusion-weighted MR imaging and light electron microscopic study. *Radiology* 1993;189:439–48.
46. Sevick RJ, Kucharczyk J, Mintorovitch J, Moseley ME, Derugin N, Norman D. Diffusion-weighted MR imaging and T_2-weighted MR imaging in acute cerebral ischemia: comparison and correlation with histopathology. *Acta Neurochirurgica* 1990;51(Suppl):210–12.
47. Minematsu K, Li L, Fisher M, Sotak CH, Davis MA, Fiandaca MS. Diffusion weighted magnetic resonance imaging: rapid and quantitative detection of focal brain ischemia. *Neurology* 1992;42:235–40.
48. Dereski MO, Chopp M, Knight RA, Chen H, Garcia JH. Focal cerebral ischemia in the rat: temporal profile of neutrophil responses. *Neurosci Res Commun* 1992;11:179.86.
49. Garcia JH, Yoshida Y, Chen H, Li Y, Zhang ZG, Lian J, Chen S, Chopp M. Progression from ischemia injury to infarct following middle cerebral artery occlusion in the rat. *Am J Pathol* 1993;142:623–35.
50. Knight RA, Dereski MO, Helpern JA, Ordidge RJ, Chopp M. MRI assessment of evolving focal cerebral ischemia: comparison with histopathology in rate. *Stroke* 1994;25:1252–62.

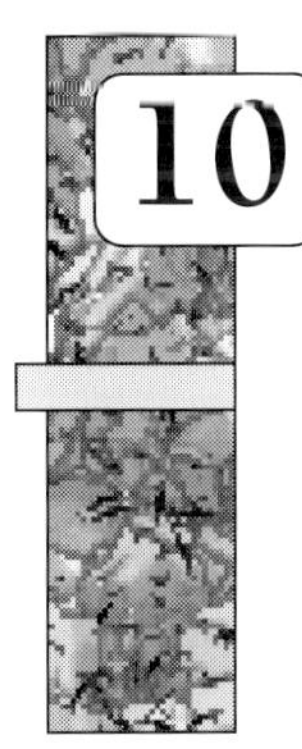

Mechanisms of Injury and Repair in Traumatic Brain Injury

Donald G. Stein, M.D., and Robin L. Roof, Ph.D.

Traumatic injury to the nervous system is not a unitary event. Rather it is a cascade of primary and secondary destructive events that can alter structure and function throughout the central nervous system (1,2). The initial impact may result in tearing, shearing, or otherwise mechanically deforming nervous tissue, especially axons and microvessels (3). In the case of trauma, the impact itself usually produces a certain amount of irreversible damage resulting in the loss of neurons, capillaries, and glial cells (4). After the initial injury, a cascade of secondary pathological reactions then produces more damage leading to neuronal loss at sites quite distant from the impact zone (5). These reactions include the excessive release of neurotransmitters and excitatory amino acids such as glutamate; intracellular calcium overload; activation of the arachidonic acid cascade; and the induction of free radical-induced lipid peroxidation. Many of the biochemical processes are interactive so they create positive feedback loops leading to distal injury (6). Within the first few hours the destructive processes produce breakdown of the blood–brain barrier, the formation of edema (6), further neuronal loss, and concomitant cognitive and functional impairments. Developing the appropriate pharmacological strategies for improving the recovery of function after brain damage requires an understanding of the multifactorial nature of the pathological changes that occur early in the process and that may continue to unfold for weeks or months. The selection of treatment would then depend considerably on which aspect or phase of the injury process must be modified in order to enhance functional recovery.

Attempts to improve recovery of function following traumatic brain injury (TBI) can be targeted to "undoing the damage," that is, promoting regeneration of nerve cells or their terminals, or preventing toxic and damaging events as they begin to unfold. Although damaged cells in the peripheral nervous system are able to elongate their injured axons and establish successful restoration of connectivity and function, the ability of central nervous system neurons to do so is very limited (7). Under most conditions, when a neuron in the adult central nervous system dies, it is not replaced.

There have been a number of attempts to devise ways of facilitating axonal and dendritic regeneration in the CNS, including the implantation of peripheral nerve tissue

(8,9,10) to provide the tips of the damaged axons with growth promoting factors (7). In some cases, axons treated in this manner have been shown to regenerate over substantial distances (9,11). For example, segments of sciatic nerve grafted into the transected spinal cord to serve as bridges have been successfully innervated by CNS axons (12,13). However, the regenerating axons do not generally grow much beyond the ends of these grafts (14). The regeneration that does occur is insufficient to restore normal amounts of interneuronal connectivity (14) and therefore there is only limited, if any, functional recovery. One reason that axons may show only limited regeneration is that non-neuronal cells such as the oligodendrocyte and astrocytes can secrete molecules that stop growth cone activity and actively inhibit the establishment of new cell-to-cell contacts causing axons to retract and die (15).

Another strategy for promoting the reconstruction of the injured nervous system is through the implantation of fetal tissue grafts. Grafting of various types of tissue (brain, spinal cord, and adrenal medulla) into the brains of patients is currently being used as treatment for Parkinson's disease and despite a number of concerns it is being proposed as therapy for TBI (16,17). Initially it was thought that embryonic brain tissue grafts would form interconnections with the host brain and thus "replace" neurons that were lost or damaged as a result of brain trauma or disease. In general, it is difficult, if not impossible, to restore the original point to point connections (18,19). Indeed, the formation of inappropriate or anomalous connections have been shown to be very detrimental. For example, Buzsaki et al. have reported that aberrant connections following hippocampal grafts can produce both physiologic and behavioral seizure induction (20). The benefits of grafts in many cases may not be due to regeneration or restoration of the normal neuronal connections, but instead tissue grafts may exert their effects through alternate mechanisms such as providing neurotransmitter replacement or trophic support (21,22). For example, Bankiewicz et al. (23) suggested that both nondopaminergic grafts and reactive astrocytes could secrete trophic factors that stimulate neuronal sprouting in the host brain. Additionally, neural grafts are capable of secreting trophic factors that promote cell survival and enhance neurite outgrowth (24). Such factors are also produced by the brain in response to injury (25). In fact, "wound extract" has been shown to facilitate the survival of some neuronal grafts (26).

Although injured or killed neurons are not replaced in nature, the CNS does have a mechanism by which it can replace some of the synaptic inputs that are lost after brain injury. When neurons die, their target cells are deprived of their normal presynaptic input. In some cases, remaining adjacent neurons will form new synapses to replace those that were lost. This process is called "reactive sprouting" or "reactive synaptogenesis" (25). Reactive synaptogenesis has been studied most extensively in the dentate gyrus of the hippocampal formation (27). In the dentate gyrus after ipsilateral entorhinal ablation, sprouting terminals from undamaged septal, commissural/associational, and contralateral entorhinal neurons occupy denervated postsynaptic sites in the outer molecular layer (25,27). It should be emphasized that reactive synaptogenesis does not replace original circuitry, but rather results in an increase in the residual input (25). The benefits of reactive synaptogenesis are highly debated (25,28). In some cases, reactive synaptogenesis has been reported to facilitate recovery of performance

(27,29,30,31). The study most often cited as supporting this argument is that by Loesche and Stewart (27). In this experiment rats learned a food motivated alternation task and then were given unilateral entorhinal cortex lesions. Within one week after injury, axonal sprouting from cells in the contralateral intact entorhinal cortex could be observed. The authors reported that the time course for recovery from the behavioral deficit paralleled the time course for the sprouting. They suggested that the new connections were mediating the recovery of spatial alternation behavior (27). However, it has also been demonstrated that behavioral recovery can occur even after bilateral entorhinal cortex lesions, in which sprouting does not occur because the neuronal pathways and target areas involved are themselves destroyed (32). Additionally, it has also been argued that reactive synaptogenesis can interfere with functional recovery either by introducing abnormal connections with the deafferented tissue (25,33), or by competing for sites with intact projections (25). Thus, if the anomalous projections were to gain the site and replace the normal contacts, the resulting behavior might also become anomalous and abnormal as well.

In some cases of compensatory sprouting after CNS lesions, the picture that emerges is very complex. For example, Fritschy and Grzanna (34) demonstrated that a noradrenergic neurotoxin (DSP-4) could produce substantial neuronal loss in the locus coeruleus. These investigators examined the degeneration and the compensatory response to this injury over a period of sixteen months after the lesion. First of all, the degeneration and regenerative response to the injury continued to take place over the course of one year. In some of the structures normally innervated by the locus coeruleus there was, indeed, marked regeneration of the LC neurons, but there was virtually none in the brainstem, cerebellum, and spinal cord—areas that normally have strong projections from the LC. Additionally, there was marked hyperinnervation in the hippocampus and frontal cortex by twelve months after the injury.

Although Fritschy and Grzanna did not perform any behavioral evaluations on their animals, it is unlikely that the markedly abnormal regeneration (hyperinnervation in the HC and FC and no reinnervation in critical brainstem regions) would have led to functional recovery at the behavioral level (20). It is also interesting to note that the processes of hyperinnervation can take up to over one year to develop. Since most investigations of functional recovery take place within a few weeks after injury, the long-term detrimental consequences of the abnormal regeneration might not be seen. Perhaps it is also important here to emphasize the need for very long-term clinical follow-up studies (i.e., many years) in patients who are given trophic factors to promote neuronal regeneration after CNS injury. In the early stages there might well be functional benefits observed which could then deteriorate as hyperinnervation or anomalous growth proceeded.

It has been demonstrated that neurite promoting factors are associated with the sprouting phenomenon (25). In light of the possible detrimental effects of axonal sprouting and its effects on functional recovery, the use of trophic factors to promote reactive sprouting should be approached with caution. In fact, under some circumstances, better functional recovery might be obtained with treatments that involve the inhibition of the sprouting response (25).

While research on promoting regenerative repair continues to generate considerable interest, another major focus in recovery of function research lies in attempts to interfere with, or limit, the pathological events that occur in early stages after brain injury. As mentioned previously, a significant amount of damage can result from the initial cascade of neurochemical and pathophysiologic events that follow TBI (5,6,35).

There are several advantages to the strategy of preventing the cascade of cytotoxicity. First, the fact that some secondary events do not occur immediately after a TBI incident allows the opportunity for pharmacologic intervention to prevent or attenuate the secondary damage. Second, reducing the pathological complications following brain injury is less likely to produce detrimental effects, while the same cannot be said for attempts to produce regeneration and sprouting of new connections. Third, by reducing free radical damage, edema formation, and glial scarring, many cells otherwise destined for death may be rescued, thereby preventing the need for strategies aimed at neuronal regeneration.

Recent research has demonstrated that neurologic outcome can be improved with pharmacologic treatment aimed at modifying secondary injury processes. By monitoring the levels of excitatory amino acids with intracerebral microdialysis techniques, it has been shown that TBI causes the excessive release of glutamate and aspartate within moments of the insult (36,37,38). High levels of amino acids can be excitotoxic to nerve tissue even at a considerable distance from the zone of initial impact (39,40,41,42). When excitatory amino acid neurotransmitters are released and activate NMDA and AMPA receptors, there is an increased influx of calcium and sodium into neurons and glia, leading to edema, vacuolization, and eventual cell death (43,44,45).

To prevent this injury cascade, NMDA receptor antagonists have been used to reduce the effects of excitatory amino acid transmitter release [for review see (35)]. There are a number of both competitive and noncompetitive receptor antagonists that seem to protect against cell death associated with cerebral ischemia and traumatic injury. For example, MK-801, a noncompetitive NMDA antagonist, can attenuate trauma-induced cerebral edema (46,47,48) and improve neurologic outcome (46,47). Unfortunately, MK-801 has also been associated with negative affects, including cytotoxicity (49,50). Some workers have reduced neuronal loss by inhibiting the release of excitatory amino acids after TBI. For example, a voltage dependent sodium channel blocker, BW1003C87, has been shown to block glutamate release *in vitro* (51,52), and *in vivo* (52,53). The intracellular accumulation of calcium due to processes other than excitotoxicity is also associated with neuronal death (6). Increased intracellular concentrations of calcium provoke an attack on the cell membrane by calcium-activated proteases and lipases and will also induce the formation of pathogenic compounds from the breakdown of arachidonic acid (6,35).

Many studies using calcium channel antagonists report improved outcome following ischemic injury [for review see (35)], but their effectiveness after TBI is less obvious. A few experimental studies have shown some beneficial effects of calcium channel blockers such as nimodipine (54), SNX-111 (55), but not (S)-emopamil (56,57); however, the latter is reportedly effective in models of ischemia (58). Additionally, clinical trials of the calcium antagonists nicardipine and nimodipine did not benefit recovery of function (59,60). Since TBI is often followed by ischemia (61), calcium overload may nonetheless be an important event to monitor and control. Additionally, because ischemia has been said to occur very early after TBI (61), successful monitoring should be begun as soon as possible after the incident.

Intracellular calcium accumulation stimulates the activation of the arachidonic acid cascade. Subsequently, arachidonic acid breakdown produces the eicosanoid metabolites, thromboxane A_2, prostaglandins, and leukotrienes (62,63), which are inflammatory and cause further cerebral edema. These substances are associated with negative outcome in experimental models of cerebral edema (64,65) and brain injury [for review see (35)]. Arachidonic acid by-products also contribute to the formation of free radicals and increased lipid peroxidation in cell membranes (6), while substances that block portions of the arachidonic acid cascade have been beneficial in some experimental brain injury models. For example, cyclooxygenase inhibitors such as ibuprofen, meclofenamic acid, and indomethacin can reduce ischemia (66,67,68), improve cerebral metabolism (69), and enhance the return of neurologic functions (70).

As mentioned before, the activation of the arachidonic acid cascade stimulates the generation of oxygen free radicals (35). Free radicals then cause the lipid peroxidation of membrane phospholipids and the oxidation of cellular proteins (6,71). Free radical induced lipid peroxidation results in compromise of the blood–brain barrier, causes edema, and kills neurons and glia (70). A variety of free radical scavengers and antioxidants have been assessed in various injury models and many have been associated with functional and morphological recovery (72–79). In our laboratory we examined the effects of α-tocopherol on recovery of function after bilateral frontal cortex aspiration in rats. We found that intracerebral administration of α-tocopherol enhanced recovery of spatial learning, blocked retrograde degeneration in the thalamus, and reduced cerebral edema (80). Other researchers observed that α-tocopherol reduced brain swelling (81), brain edema, reactive gliosis, lipid peroxidation, and neuronal necrosis (82).

Free radical *scavengers* have also been assessed in the treatment of CNS injury. The glucocorticoid steroid methylprednisolone is reported to have significant antioxidant capabilities and can enhance neurologic outcome in spinal cord trauma (83,84,85). The doses required to obtain beneficial results, however, are problematic because they can cause a number of incapacitating side effects (86), including hyperglycemia, catabolic states, and increased incidence of serious infections (87,88,89). Recently, a series of 21-aminosteroid compounds with structural resemblance to methylprednisolone, but without the glucocorticoid activity, have been developed and tested by Upjohn Pharmaceutical. These new compounds may have greater antioxidant efficacy than methylprednisolone and fewer side effects (90,91).

Many of the secondary injury processes discussed thus far result in the compromise of the blood–brain barrier and the formation of cerebral edema. Brain edema itself has serious consequences, including pathological intracranial swelling leading to neuronal loss and eventually death (92). The secondary neuronal death resulting from such events can be responsible for a larger proportion of cell loss than the initial injury itself (93). However, if focal cerebral edema is rapidly reduced, residual fluid and electrolytes are eventually removed and the neuropil is restored to a relatively normal state. The presence of edema may be caused initially by lipid peroxidation, the arachidonic acid cascade, or other secondary processes. Additionally, as mentioned earlier, formation of edema may stimulate a positive feedback situation in which these destructive processes are enhanced (6,35).

Over the last several years, our laboratory has published a series of papers demonstrating that following bilateral contusion injury of the frontal cortex, progesterone is capable of reducing edema (94,95), improving the integrity of the blood–brain barrier (96), and reducing free radical induced lipid peroxidation of membranes (97). The posttraumatic treatment with progesterone also reduced retrograde neuronal degeneration in the thalamus and improved the recovery of cognitive performance in spatial learning tasks (98). Our initial finding showed that females have less cerebral edema than males after a cortical contusion of the frontal cortex (97). Subsequent experiments demonstrated that this gender difference was due to the presence of higher levels of progesterone in the female (94,97). We subsequently were able to show that treatment with progesterone confers the same protection to males as was found in females (94). These results are shown in Figure 10-1A. Beneficial effects were seen when the progesterone was given before, as well as after, the injury. Since a causal factor in vasogenic edema is the breakdown of the blood–brain barrier, we examined the effect of progesterone injections on the integrity of the BBB. We found that three days after contusions, male rats given progesterone exhibited a more intact BBB (96). Our research also demonstrated that contused brains from progesterone-treated rats contained less of a free radical lipid peroxidation breakdown product (8 isoprostane), than contused, non-treated rats (95). This can be taken to suggest that there had been less free radical associated membrane breakdown in the progesterone-treated rats. As mentioned previously, progesterone treatments following bilateral medial contusions also result in a reduced cell loss in the medial dorsal nucleus of the thalamus, as shown in Figure 10-1B, as well as improved cognitive performance, as shown in Figure 10-2 (96). These data can be taken to demonstrate that progesterone has potential as a treatment for TBI, and also exemplifies the interactive nature of these secondary processes, i.e., treatment of each secondary process can lead to reductions in the severity of the other processes.

In conclusion, it is safe to say that over the last ten years there has been an explosion of research on neurotrauma and on the means to treat its consequences as early as possible in the injury process. Although all of the mechanisms and manifestations of head trauma are not yet fully understood, it is now clear that the term "CNS injury" represents a multitude of processes that continue to unfold long after the initial events leading to neuronal loss have subsided. Stabilization of the head-injured patient is clearly the first objective in emergency care, but the need for immediate pharmacologic intervention designed to block the cascade of cytotoxic events that will cause further neuronal degeneration cannot be overemphasized. The immediate rescue of neurons and their complement of sustaining glial cells may be the first step required to maintain functional capacity. The stimulation of specific patterns of neuronal regeneration in an attempt to replace the loss of normal connections between different brain areas is also an essential area of research. However, the attempts to promote regeneration to reestablish previously damaged pathways must be undertaken with great care if one is to proceed to the clinic with this approach. As mentioned earlier, the creation of anomalous pathways and the hyperinnervation of previously denervated

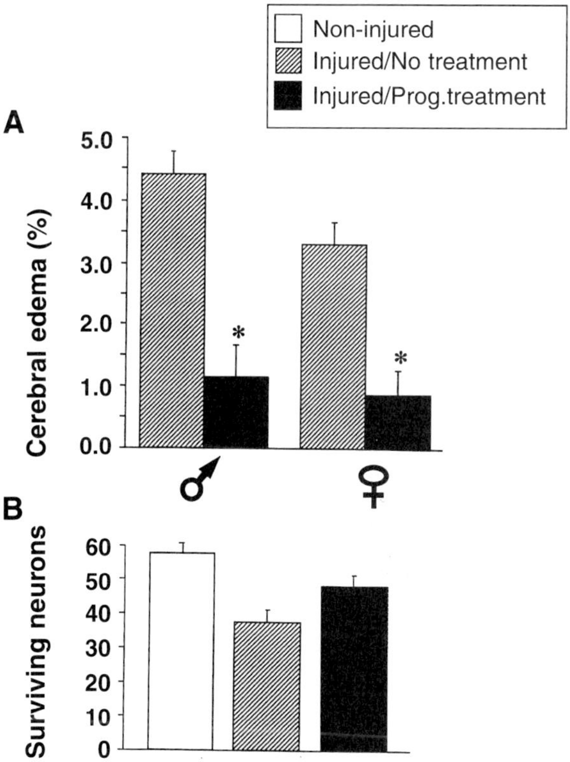

Figure 10-1. (A) Cerebral edema in cortically contused male and female rats given progesterone or oil injections. Edema is expressed as percent increase in water content in injured compared to non-injured tissue. (B) Neuronal density in the medial dorsal nucleus of the thalamus in non-injured or cortically contused male rats given progesterone or oil injections.

areas may actually prevent, rather than restore, functional recovery. The process itself may take very extended periods of time, which would mean that multi-year, long-term follow-up studies of patients undergoing experimental therapy with trophic factors is essential. Molecular biological and pharmacological research is certainly the *sine qua non* for progress in this fundamental area of medicine, but it is also important to recognize and emphasize again that not every change at the molecular or cellular level of analysis will necessarily be beneficial to the patient. This is why careful behavioral and functional studies must be done in conjunction with the physiological. The production of trophic factors, the increase in neurotransmitter levels, or the stimulation of new pathways must be carefully assessed in the laboratory to determine if such changes are beneficial, detrimental, or of no consequence to the functioning organism in both the short- and long-term. Only in this manner can the risks of novel treatments be reduced and the improvements in the quality of life for the victims of head injury be assured.

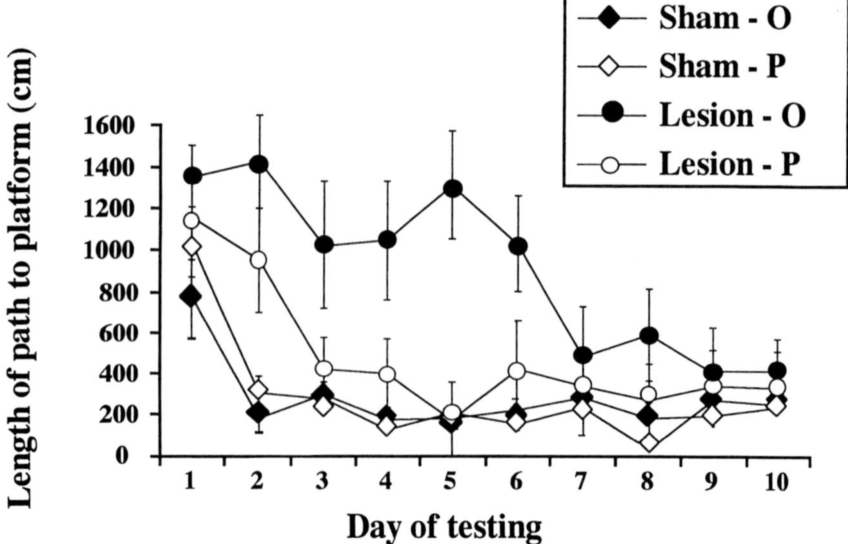

Figure 10-2. Water maze performance. Mean length of path to platform in cm on each day of testing for oil or progesterone treated male rats after cortical contusion or sham surgery. Bars indicate standard errors.

References

1. Livingston KE. *A neurosurgical blindspot.* 3rd International Congress of Neurological Surgery, Amsterdam, Excerpta Medica 1967.

2. Miller JD. Head injury and brain ischemia—implications for therapy. *Brit J Anaesthesiol* 1985;57:120–30.

3. Povlishock JT. Traumatically induced axonal injury: pathogenesis and pathobiological implications. *Brain Pathology* 1992;2:1–12.

4. White RJ, Likavec MJ. The diagnosis and initial management of head injury. *New Engl J Med* 1992;327(21):1507–11.

5. Nieto-Sampedro M, et al. Brain injury causes a time dependent increase in neurotrophic activity in the lesion site. *Science* 1982;217:860–61.

6. Hall ED, Traystman RJ. *Current concepts: secondary tissue damage after CNS injury.* The Upjohn Company, 1993.

7. Bray GM, et al. (eds.). *Regeneration of axons from the central nervous system of adult rats.* Progress in Brain Research. Elsevier, 1987.

8. Richardson PM, et al. Axons from CNS neurons regenerate into PNS grafts. *Nature* 1980;284:264–65.

9. David S, Aguayo AJ. Axonal elongation into PNS 'bridges' after CNS injury in adult rats. *Science* 1981;214:931–33.

10. Aguayo AJ. Axonal regeneration from injured neurons in the adult mammalian central nervous system. *Synaptic plasticity and remodeling.* New York, Guilford Press, 1985:457–83.

11. Benfey M, Aguayo AJ. Extensive elongation of axons in rat brain into peripheral nerve grafts. *Nature* 1982;296:150–52.

12. Friedman B, Aguayo AJ. Injured neurons in the olfactory bulb of the adult rat grow axons along grafts of peripheral nerve. *J Neurosci* 1985;5:1616–25.

13. Schwab ME, Thoenen H. Dissociated neurons regenerate into sciatic but not optic nerve transplants in culture irrespective of neurotrophic factors. *J Neurosci* 1985;5:2415–23.

14. Freed WJ, et al. Promoting functional plasticity in the damaged nervous system. *Science* 1985;227:1544–52.

15. Johnson AR. Contact inhibition in the failure of mammalian CNS axonal regeneration. *BioEssays* 1993;15:807–13.

16. Dunnett SB (ed). *Is it possible to repair the damaged prefrontal cortex by neural tissue transplantation?* Progress in Brain Research. Elsevier, 1990.

17. Stein DG. Some practical and theoretical issues concerning fetal brain tissue grafts as therapy for brain dysfunctions. *Behav Brain Sci* 1995,18:36–45.

18. Stein DG, Mufson EJ. Morphological and behavioral characteristics of embryonic brain tissue transplants in adult, brain-damaged subjects. *Cell and tissue transplantation into the adult brain.* 1987;444–65.

19. Sotelo C, Alvarado-Mallart RM. The reconstruction of cerebellar circuits. *Trends Neurosci* 1991;14:350–55.

20. Buzsaki G, et al. The grafted hippocampus: an epileptic focus. *Exp Neurol* 1989;105:10–22.

21. Labbe R, et al. Fetal brain transplants: reduction of cognitive deficits in rats with frontal cortex lesions. *Science* 1983;217:470–72.

22. Ikegami S, et al. Recovery of hippocampal cholinergic activity in AF64A treated rats. *Neurosci Lett* 1989;101:17–22.

23. Bankiewicz KS, et al. Fetal nondopaminergic neural implants in parkinsonian primates. *J Neurosurg* 1991;74:97–104.

24. Cotman CW, Kesslak JP. The role of trophic factors in behavioral recovery and integration of transplants. *Transplantation into mammalian CNS.* Elsevier, 1988:311–20.

25. Nieto-Sampedro M. Growth factor induction and order of events in CNS repair. *Pharmacological approaches to the treatment of brain and spinal cord injury.* New York, Plenum Press, 1988:301–37.

26. Nieto-Sampedro M, et al. The survival of brain transplants is enhanced by extracts from injured brain. *Proc Nat Acad Sci* 1984;1:6250–54.

27. Loesche J, Stewart O. Behavioral correlates of denervation and reinnervation of the hippocampal formation of the rat: recovery of alternation performance following unilateral entorhinal cortex lesions. *Brain Res Bull* 1977;2:31–39.

28. Finger S, Almli CR. Brain damage and neuroplasticity: mechanisms of recovery or development? *Brain Res Rev* 1985;10:177–86.

29. Rosner BS. Brain functions. *Ann Rev Psychol* 1970;21:555–94.

30. Goldberger ME, Murray M. Restitution of function and collateral sprouting in the cat spinal cord: the deafferented animal. *J Comp Neurol* 1974;158:37.

31. Scheff S, Cotman CW. Reactive synaptogenesis in the adult nervous system. *Neuronal recognition.* New York, Plenum Press, 1977: 69–108.

32. Ramirez JJ, Stein DG. Sparing and recovery of spatial alternation performance after entorhinal cortex lesions in rats. *Behav Brain Res* 1984;13:53–61.

33. Leong SK. Plasticity of cerebellar afferents after neonatal lesions in albino rats. *Neurosci Lett* 1978;7:281–89.

34. Fritschy J-M, Grzanna R. Restoration of ascending noradrenergic projections by residual locus coeruleus neurons: compensatory response to neurotoxin-induced cell death in the adult rat brain. *J Comp Neurol* 1992; 321:421–41.

35. McIntosh TK. Neurochemical sequelae of traumatic brain injury: therapeutic implications. *Cerebrovasc Brain Metab Rev* 1994;6(2):109–62.

36. Faden AI, et al. The role of excitatory amino acids and NMDA receptors in traumatic brain injury. *Science* 1989;244:798–800.

37. Katayama Y, et al. Massive increases in extracellular potassium and the indiscriminate release of glutamate following concussive brain injury. *J Neurosurg* 1990;73:889–900.

38. Palmer AM, et al. Traumatic brain injury-induced excitotoxicity assessed in a controlled cortical impact model. *J Neurochem* 1993;61:2015–24

39. Olney JW, et al. Cytotoxic effects of acidic and sulfur-containing amino acid on the infant mouse nervous system. *Exp Brain Res* 1971;14:61–76.

40. Rothman S, Olney JW. Glutamate and the pathophysiology of hypoxic ischemic brain damage. *Ann Neurol* 1986;19:105–11.

41. Olney JW, et al. MK-801 powerfully protects against N-methyl aspartate neurotoxicity. *Eur J Pharmacol* 1987;141:357–61.

42. Rothman S, Olney JW. Excitotoxicty and the NMDA receptor. *Trends in Neurosci* 1987;10:299–302.

43. Choi D. Ionic dependence of glutamate neurotoxicity. *J Neurosci* 1987;7:369–79.

44. Choi D, et al. Glutamate neurotoxicity in cortical cell culture. *J Neurosci* 1987;7:357–68.

45. Choi D. Calcium-mediated neurotoxicity: relationship to specific channel types and its role in ischemic damage. *Trends in Neurosci* 1989;11:21–26.

46. McIntosh TK, et al. (ed.). *The NMDA receptor antagonist MK-801 prevents edema and restores magnesium homeostasis after traumatic brain injury in the rat.* Frontiers in excitatory amino acid research. New York, Alan Liss, 1988.

47. McIntosh TK, et al. Effects of N-methyl-D-aspartate receptor blocker MK-801 on neurological function after experimental brain injury. *J Neurotrauma* 1989;6:247–59.

48. Shapira Y, et al. Protective effects of MK-801 in experimental brain injury. *J Cereb Blood Flow Metab* 1990;8:962–68.

49. Olney JW, et al. MK-801 prevents hyperbaric ischemic neuron degeneration in infant rat brain. *J Neurosci* 1989;9:1701–1704.

50. Sharp F, et al. MK-801 and ketamine induce heat shock protein HSP72 in injured neurons in posterior cingulate and retrosplenial cortex. *Ann Neurol* 1991;30:801–809.

51. Leach MJ, et al. Lamotrigine, a novel potential antiepileptic drug: 2. Neurochemical studies on the mechanism of action. *Epilepsia* 1986;27:490–97.

52. Meldrum BS, et al. Reduction of glutamate release and protection against ischemic brain damage by BW 1003C87. *Brain Res* 1992;593:1–6.

53. Graham SH, et al. Limiting ischemic injury by inhibition of excitatory amino acid release. *J Cereb Blood Flow Metab* 1993;13:88–97.

54. Levere TE, et al. Recovery of function after brain damage—the benefits of diets supplemented with the calcium channel blocker nimodipine. *Psychobiology* 1992;20(3): 219–22.

55. Bodie H, et al. A selective N-channel calcium blocker attenuates the injury-induced accumulation of calcium following experimental traumatic brain injury. *J Neurotrauma* 1993;10:161.

56. Okiyama K, et al. Effects of calcium channel blocker (S)-emopamil on regional cerebral edema and neurobehavioral function after experimental brain injury. *J Neurosurg* 1992;77:607–15.

57. Okiyama K, et al. Evaluation of a novel calcium channel blocker, (S)-emopamil, on regional cerebral edema and neurobehavioral function after experimental brain injury. *J Neurosurg* 1992;77(4): 607–15.

58. Okiyama K, et al. (S)-emopamil attenuates regional cerebral blood flow reduction following experimental brain injury. *J Neurotrauma* 1994;11:83–95.

59. Compton JS, et al. A double blind placebo controlled trial of the calcium entry blocking drug nicardipine in the treatment of vasospasm following severe head injury. *Brit J Neurosurg* 1990;4:9–16.

60. Teasdale G. A randomized trial of nimodipine in severe head injury. HIT 1. *J Neurotrauma* 1991;37:S545–50.

61. Bouma GJ, et al. Cerebral circulation and metabolism after severe traumatic brain injury: the elusive role of ischemia. *J Neurosurg* 1991;75:685–93.

62. Wolfe L, Coceani F. The role of prostaglandins in the central nervous system. *Ann Rev Physiol* 1979;41:669–84.

63. Leslie JB, Watkins WD. Eicosanoids in the central nervous system. *J Neurosurg* 1985;63:659–68.

64. Chan P, Fishman R. Transient formation of superoxide radicals in polyunsaturated fatty acid induced brain swelling. *J Neurochem* 1980;35:1004–1007.

65. Black KL, Hoff JT. Leukotrienes increase blood–brain barrier permeability following intrapparenchymal injections in rats. *Ann Neurol* 1985;18:349–51.

66. Hallenbeck J, Furlow T. Prostaglandin 1-2 and indomethacin prevent impairment of postischemic brain reperfusion in the dog. *Stroke* 1979;10:629–37.

67. Hallenbeck JT, et al. Combined PGI2, indomethacin and heparin improve recovery after spinal trauma in cats. *J Neurosurg* 1983;58:749–54.

68. Grice S, et al. Ibuprofen improves cerebral blood flow after global cerebral ischemia in dogs. *Stroke* 1987;18:787–91.

69. Pappius HM, Wolfe L. Functional disturbances in brain following injury. *Neurochem Res* 1983;8:63–72.

70. Hall E. Beneficial effects of acute intravenous ibuprofen on neurologic recovery of head-injured mice: comparison of cyclooxygenase inhibition with inhibition of thromboxane A2 synthetase or 5-lipoxygenase. *J Neurotrauma* 1985;2:75–83.

71. Kontos HA. Oxygen radicals in cerebral ischemia. *Cerebrovascular diseases—sixteenth research (Princeton) conference.* New York, Plenum Press, 1989:365–71.

72. Yamamoto M, et al. A possible role of lipid peroxidation in cellular damage caused by cerebral ischemia and the protective effect of α-tocopherol administration. *Stroke* 1983;14:977 82.

73. Yoshida S, et al. Postischemic cerebral lipid peroxidation in vitro: modification by dietary vitamin E. *J Neurochem* 1985;44:1593–1601.

74. Chan P, et al. Protective effects of liposome-entrapped superoxide dimutase on posttraumatic brain edema. *Ann Neurol* 1987;21:540–47.

75. Abe K, et al. Strong attenuation of ischemic and postischemic brain edema in rats by a novel free radical scavenger. *Stroke* 1988;19:480–85.

76. Sakaki S, et al. Free radical reaction and biological defense mechanism in the pathogenesis and prolonged vasospasm in experimental subarachnoid hemorrhage. *J Cereb Blood Flow Metab* 1988;8:1–8.

77. Clifton G, et al. Effect of Dl α-tocopheryl succinate and polyethylene glycol on performance tests after fluid percussion brain injury. *J Neurotrauma* 1989;6:71–81.

78. Hall ED, et al. Correlation between attenuation of posttraumatic spinal cord ischemia and preservation of tissue vitamin E by the 21-aminosteriod U74006F: evidence for an in vivo antioxidant mechanism. *J Neurotrauma* 1989;6(3):169–76.

79. Bracken MB, et al. Methylprednisolone or naloxone treatment after acute spinal cord injury. *J Neurosurg* 1992;76:23–31.

80. Stein DG, et al. Intracerebral administration of Alpha-Tocopherol-containing liposomes facilitates behavioral recovery in rats with bilateral lesions of the frontal cortex. *J Neurotrauma* 1991;8(4):281–92.

81. Yoshida S, et al. Compression induced brain edema: modification by prior depletion and supplementation of vitamin E. *J Cereb Blood Flow Metab* 1983;33:166–72.

82. Willimore LJ, Rubin JJ. Antiperoxidant pretreatment and iron-induced epileptiform discharges in the rat: EEG and histopathologic studies. *Neurol* 1981;31:63–69.

83. Young W, et al. Pharmacological therapy of acute spinal cord injury: studies with high dose methylprednisolone and naloxone. *Clin Neurosurg* 1988;34:675–97.

84. Holtz A, et al. Effects of methylprednisolone on motor function and spinal cord blood flow after spinal cord compression in rats. *Acta Neurol Scand* 1990;82:68–73.

85. Bracken MB, et al. A randomized, controlled trial of methylprednisolone or naloxone in the treatment of acute spinal cord injury. *New Engl J Med* 1992;322:1405–11.

86. Hall ED. Lipid antioxidants in acute central nervous system injury. *Ann Emerg Med* 1993;22(6): 1022–26.

87. DeMaria EJ, et al. Septic complications of corticosteroid administration after central nervous system trauma. *Ann Surg* 1985;202:248–52.

88. Robertson CS, et al. Steroid administration and nitrogen excretion in the head-injured patient. *J Neurosurg* 1985;63:203–209.

89. Deutschman CS, et al. Physiological and metabolic response to isolated closed head injury. Part 2. Effects of steroids on metabolism. Potentiation of protein wasting and abnormalities of substrate utilization. *J Neurosurg* 1987;66:388–95.

90. Hall ED, et al. New pharmacological treatments for spinal cord trauma. *J Neurotrauma* 1988;5:81–89.

91. Braughler JM, et al. The 21-aminosteroids: potent inhibitors of lipid peroxidation for the treatment of central nervous system trauma and ischemia. *Drugs Future* 1989;14:143–52.

92. Betz AL, et al. Brain edema: a classification based on blood–brain barrier integrity. *Cerebrovasc Brain Metab Rev* 1989;1:133–54.

93. Cervos-Navarro J, Lafuente JV. Traumatic brain injuries: structural changes. *J Neurol Sci* 1991;103:S3–S14.

94. Roof RL, et al. Progesterone treatment attenuates brain edema following contusion injury in male and female rats. *Restorative Neurology and Neuroscience* 1992;4:425–27.

95. Roof RL, et al. Gender influences outcome of brain injury: progesterone plays protective role. *Brain Res* 1993;607:333–36.

96. Roof RL, et al. Progesterone facilitates cognitive recovery and reduces secondary neuronal loss following cortical contusion injury in male rats. *Exp Neurol* 1994;129:64–69.

97. Roof RL, et al. Progesterone reduces free radical induced membrane peroxidation following traumatic brain injury. *Soc Neuro Abs* 1993;20:191.

98. Roof RL, et al. (1994). Progesterone reduces BBB damage following bilateral, medial frontal contusion. *J Neurosurg,* submitted.

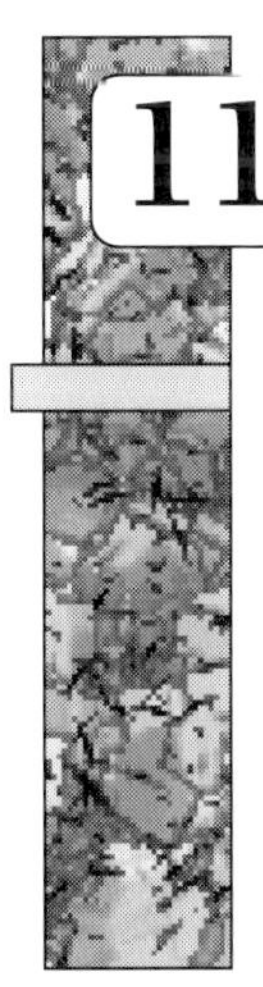

11

Pattern of Brain Damage in a Traumatic Brain Injury Model: Noradrenergic Pharmacotherapy Promotes Recovery of Function

Dennis M. Feeney, Ph.D.

The remarkable expansion of research on traumatic brain injury (TBI) over the last decade has led to promising treatments for promoting functional recovery. This is in contrast to the hopeless viewpoint prevalent just twenty-five years ago. Basic research into processes initiated by TBI has provided a scientific basis for pharmacotherapy. Additionally, developments in clinical imaging methods have refined diagnosis of the cerebral pathologies produced by TBI and stroke. The fusion of these disciplines has great potential, requiring collaborative efforts that will require significant increases in funding to realize the objectives of such work.

An increase in research funding is likely to produce significant financial returns to society. The need for intervention to promote recovery after TBI cannot be overemphasized. Cerebral trauma is the leading cause of permanently disabling injuries affecting 30,000 to 50,000 Americans each year. Health care costs and lost income for patients with permanent disabilities due to trauma are enormous (1,2), and the emotional consequences for those individuals and their families are incalculable. Direct financial costs of TBI are greater than those of stroke or degenerative diseases, which primarily afflict the elderly, whereas TBI primarily strikes the young (1). Brain-injured patients very often require prolonged, costly, and labor-intensive care; the average per case treatment cost for the first year alone following severe TBI, excluding rehabilitation expenditures, was calculated in 1990 as $105,380 (2). For most severe TBI cases the costs of rehabilitation continue for many years. Accelerating recovery from brain injury could hasten the return of individuals to an active life and reduce the enormous financial and personal costs of a neurologic disability. The results of our investigations are relevant to clinicians attempting to interpret imaging studies of brain injured patients. Increased understanding of the pathophysiological mechanisms underlying injury will improve diagnosis and patient care.

Modeling Pathological Sequelae of Traumatic Brain Injury

This chapter is limited to coverage of three aspects of TBI pathology and some mention of related topics in stroke, since the issues are well covered in many neuropathology texts (3). The focus of this discussion will be on laboratory modeling of some pathological and behavioral consequences of TBI in human beings and their experimental treatments. Following a focal impact trauma to the rat sensorimotor cortex (SMCX), there is a cascade of neuropathological sequelae. Of these, three qualitatively different types of pathological categories have been studied in the weight drop TBI model using the rat. The three pathologies and their possible pharmacological treatments to be discussed include: first, a focal contusion of SMCX, which is a slow developing pannecrotic cyst near the impact site. I will review data indicating that the very slow evolution of a cortical contusion over a period of weeks leads to a fluid-filled cyst which engulfs many neurons that survived the initial trauma and other early pathological events. Such very delayed neuronal death has been described in a stroke model (6) but has received very little attention. Second, selective neuronal injury (SNI), the death of certain vulnerable neurons adjacent to intact cells following brain injury. In the weight drop model used in my laboratory (4), SNI is confined to ipsilateral structures, most notably the hilar and the usually insult-resistant CA3 hippocampal regions. SNI is also observed in the dorsolateral striatum, medial geniculate (pars magnocellular division), ventral basal complex of the thalamus, and the thalamic reticular nucleus. Study of the latter structure has just begun (Feeney and Weisend, note added in proof). Third, remote functional depression (RFD) or *diaschisis*, a term denoting functional perturbations in structurally intact areas remote from the locus of morphological damage. Such changes are thought to result from either excess or absence of neuronal input to the cells as a result of the injury. I will also review laboratory data from pharmacology studies of a promising short-term therapy that enhances physical therapy and can be initiated weeks after brain injury. Other data indicate pharmacological increase of α-noradrenergic synaptic activity alleviates symptoms of focal brain injury by an effect on RFD. The clinical data pertaining to our experimental observations of beneficial or harmful effects of drugs respectively increasing or decreasing α-noradrenergic synapses activity is reviewed by Goldstein in this volume (7) and by others elsewhere (8). These processes evolve at different rates, are associated with different symptoms, and respond to different treatments. Additionally, mention of other posttraumatic sequelae, including ischemia, hyperemia, hemorrhage, hydrocephalus, and seizures, are briefly noted in this review.

Weight-Drop Traumatic Brain Injury Model

These well-documented reactions all occur in the weight drop TBI model (4) and so provide the investigator an opportunity to examine potential therapies for different types of injuries and associated symptoms within the same animal. The most prominent feature of severe TBI in human beings is the presence of multiple injuries; especially diffuse axonal injury (DAI), contusions, subarachnoid hemorrhage, ischemia, and hyperemia with SNI in particularly vulnerable structures such as the hippocampus. We acknowledge that no current model will reliably reproduce all of these events. The purpose of a TBI model is to isolate and reproduce a subset of physiological events and/or processes of the more complex, multiple consequences of the to-be-modeled event. The method used to produce the events and processes is irrelevant. However, the biophysics of TBI and models should be studied, as some aspects of the injury may result from impact kinetics. Such modeling of impact kinetics led to the recent development of an impact model producing DAI. Performing a contralateral craniotomy and opening of the dura prior to impact trauma, simulations indicated this would result in mechanical deformation across the midline, presumably focused at the opening rather than diffusing throughout the hemisphere. Experiments using rats indicated that this produced a widespread pattern of forebrain axonal injury similar to DAI following TBI in human beings (5).

The weight drop TBI model I developed (4) produces a single contusion in SMCX, a location that is infrequent in TBI patients. However, for laboratory studies, the location is irrelevant. This site was selected because it results in readily measurable somatosensory and locomotor symptoms in the rat, remarkably similar to hemiplegia in human beings. The weight drop TBI rat model also results in "cognitive" deficits, poor performance on some learning and memory tests, especially those sensitive to hippocampal injury. Thus, using this model, treatment effects can be studied on both the contusion, hippocampal SNI, RFD, and associated symptoms.

The weight drop TBI device is illustrated in Figure 11-1. When the impact is centered on the hind limb area of the rat sensorimotor cortex (SMCX), which is relatively flat and accessible, it produces a transient contralateral hemiplegia. The lysencephalic rat cortex avoids the complications attributable to mechanical and/or blood supply alterations of processes due to convolutions of the cerebral cortex of other species. This simplification for laboratory investigations permits us to study the mechanisms of contusion. The behavioral deficit after a 400g/cm injury (20 gm weight dropped 20 cm though a vented tube onto a footplate limiting cortical penetration to 2.5 mm) in the rat is not very obvious when the animal is on a flat surface. The severe hemiplegia is revealed by placing the animal on a narrow elevated beam (4).

Contusion: A Pancellular Necrosis Evolving into a Fluid-Filled Cyst

At the site of impact, and expanding lateral but not medial, is a pancellular necrosis, the death of all cells in the area of traumatized SMCX, which is seen as a slowly growing fluid-filled cavity. The lateral expansion of the cavity into cortex not directly injured while sparing neurons under the medial traumatized cortex (9) was unexpected. Most likely this is due to the compression of cortex into the downward curve of the adjacent lateral skull and reflectance of impact forces from that rigid surface (Feeney et al., note added in proof). Also, the contralateral hemisphere may serve as a "cushion" for the medial cortex. While there is considerable variance in shape of contusions, at low impact severity it has a morphological appearance similar to cortical contusions in human beings (3). However, while in both species they are wedge-shaped, in the human they are described as an inverted wedge, whereas after mild injury in rat the apex of the wedge is at the cortical surface (see Figures 11-2 and 11-3). This may be

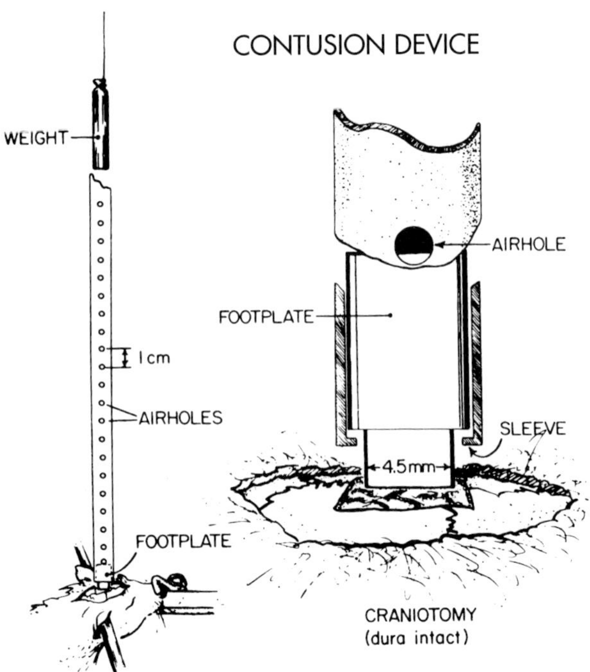

Figure 11-1. Weight drop device for producing focal contusion, selective neuronal injury in ipsilateral subcortex and remote metabolic dysfunction in structurally intact areas remote from the injuries. A 40 cm vented tube guides a falling weight onto a footplate resting on the dura. A sleeve at the tube base limits penetration into cortex to 2.5 mm. Impact force is expressed in terms of parameters, e.g., 200 g/cm injury is produced by a 20 gm weight dropped 10 cm. (*Reproduced from Feeney et al., 1981, with permission.*).

due to differences in circulation in the cortex of rat and human being. The lysencephalic rat has its cortical blood supply from radial arteries penetrating from the surface. In human beings, contusions are most often at the crest of gyri, and arteries in the depths of adjacent fissures give rise to laterally penetrating arterioles. Perhaps in human beings these provide collateral circulation to the cortical depth of injured tissue also innervated by the fragile terminals of the arteries originating from the surface. Rupture of these end arteries appears to be an important factor in the origin of contusions (4). More severe contusions in the rat have the shape of a cylinder, tapering at each end in white matter (Figure 4, Feeney et al. poster on the Internet at http://spine.unm.edu/neurosurg/sym/welcome3.html). The data from light microscopic studies indicate a slow evolution of pannecrosis expanding from this area of damage over a two-week period after TBI (4). The damage slowly progresses from scattered petechial hemorrhages in the white matter and deep cortical layers of traumatized cortex in the first hours after TBI (Figures 11-2 and 11-3A) to a cystic cavity of stable volume by thirty days (Figures 11-3B and 11-4). The continued slow

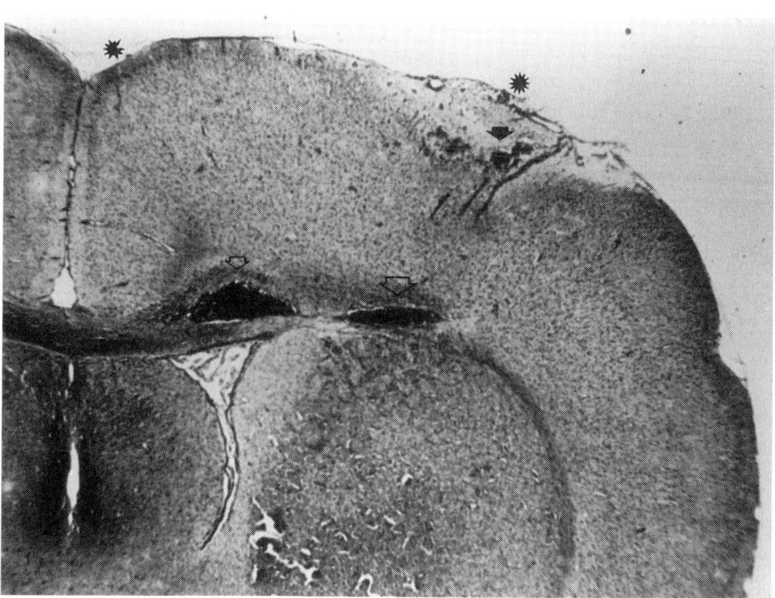

Figure 11-2. Frozen 40u, thionin stained coronal section taken 2 hours following a 200 gm/cm impact to rat SMCX. Note scattered petchial hemorrhages in injured cortex (*solid arrow*) and large hemorrhages at the cortical-callosal junction (*block arrows*), characteristic of the first hours of a contusion injury. The large hemorrhages are located where the first cavitation necrosis is observed one day after TBI illustrated in Figure 11-3A. Also in the area that will evolve into a cavity the tissue is quite pale, with occluded vessels especially at the surface near the lateral edge of the footplate (*asterisk*). Cortex immediately under the medial footplate edge (*asterisk*) survives for days following impact (9). For further discussion of neuronal survival at the impact site see the Notes Added in Proof and Poster EE0505 in the Internet symposium at http://spine.unm.edu/neurosurg/sym/welcome3.html.

expansion of the cavity may in part be related to lysosomal proteolytic enzyme activity, presumably in glial cells, on the border of the cavity as illustrated in Figure 11-4. Surprisingly, many neurons survive for at least three days in the SMCX area destined to evolve into a fluid-filled cavity depicted in Figure 11-5. Experiments using micro-dialysis measurements of neurotransmitters and metabolic products in contused cortex show an immediate and massive release of excitatory amino acids (EAA) to neurotoxic levels and indicate a disturbance of metabolism (10). Despite the direct trauma and excitotoxic events, at three days after the contusion in some regions as large as 20% of the eventual cavity, the majority of neurons still appear anatomically normal since they are not acidophilic or argyrophilic and do not appear injured (eccentric nuclei or pale cytoplasm) in thionin stained sections (9). The viability of these "normal" appearing neurons has been verified using physiological procedures. Neurons in the area of a contusion, but not an undercut lesion, remain reactive to microstimulation for up to two weeks (11), and so are also physiologically viable for a prolonged

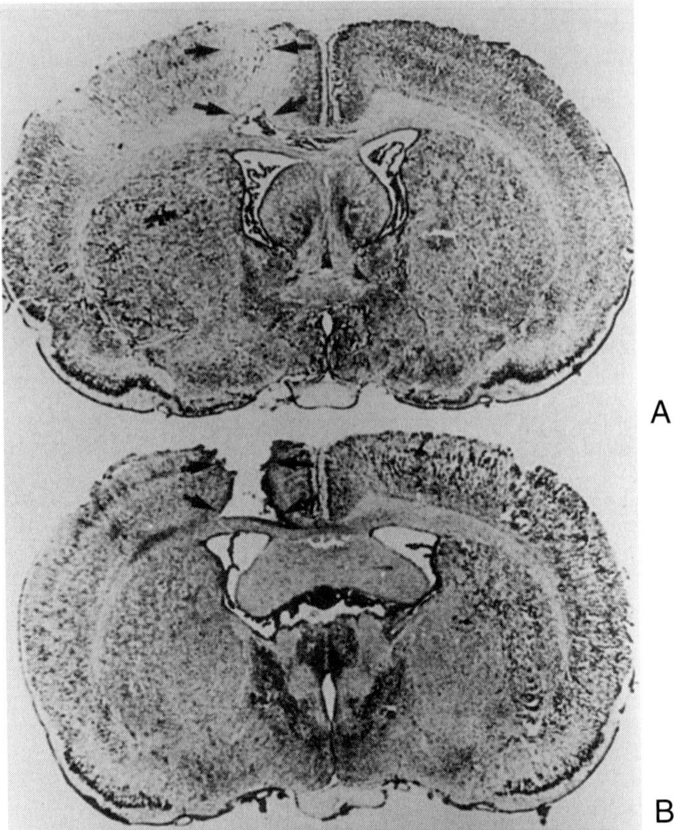

Figure 11-3. Expansion of cystic necrosis progresses slowly over weeks. At 24 hours (A) after trauma, pancellular necrotic cavitation (*arrows*) first appears at the locus of earlier hemorrhages. By 15 days (B) these expand and coalesce into a single cavity engulfing neurons surviving the impact and early secondary pathological events. Illustrations prepared as in Figure 11-2. (*Reproduced from Feeney et al., 1981, with permission.*)

time after TBI. These observations suggest a long-lasting potential for neuronal rescue in the area of an expanding contusion days after TBI. After stabilizing between two and four weeks, the extent of cortical necrosis remains relatively unchanged for months (4) but expands again in some aged animals injured in their adolescence (Feeney, unpublished observations). For a given severity of impact (e.g., 400 g/cm), there is some variance between subjects [(12) and see Figure 11-6)] and the volume of the cortical contusion is highly correlated with other behavioral and anatomical measures of TBI severity, including SNI in hippocampus, medial geniculate, and ventral basal complex. However, neuronal injury in the dorsolateral striatum after TBI is not correlated with other measures of injury severity (12). This suggests that the neuronal death in the dorsolateral striatum, which is also seen in hypoxia/ischemia, is initiated by trauma but progresses under control of factors independent of events in the other regions. Change in brain

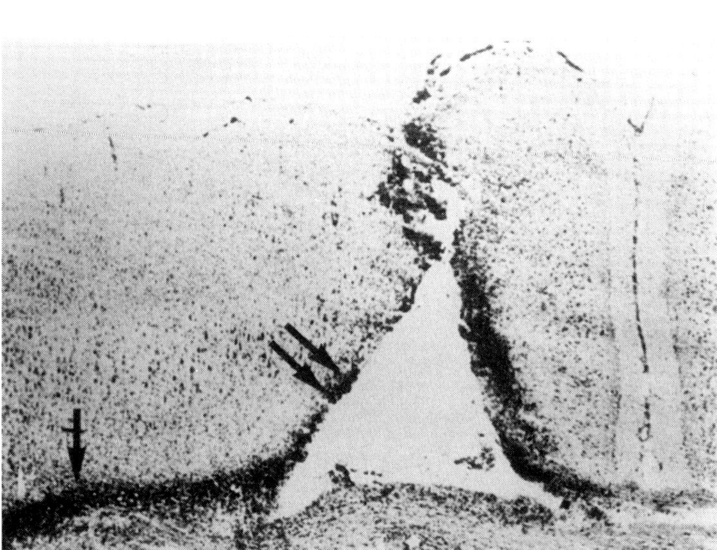

Figure 11-4. Histochemical stain for acid phosphatase indicates a marked cellular reaction of this lysosomal enzyme at the borders of a cavity (*double arrows*) 15 days after injury produced as in the previous figures. The white matter lateral to the contusion also contains intense acid phosphatse activity (*single arrow*) indicative of degenerating axons. (*Reproduced from Feeney et al., 1981, with permission.*)

temperature after TBI is a symptom of TBI severity and highly correlated with volume of the subsequent cortical contusion, body weight loss, and severity of hemiplegia (12). Thus, measurement of brain temperature five to ten minutes after injury can predict the severity of many other responses to TBI.

Although some authors consider the weight drop contusion method too variable for a good TBI model, this is an unfounded assumption. First, undue variance within any model most often depends on the surgery rather than the device. Second, there are no data to support this proposition. We measured the volume of cortical contusion after varying trauma severity using the weight drop TBI model. As illustrated in Figure 11-6, the volume of contusion is a linear function of impact force (4). We have replicated the injury volume to within one standard error in more recent studies despite changes in anesthetic (12,13). Data indicating the reproducibility of the consequences of TBI are not available for many laboratory models.

Posttraumatic Hydrocephalus

Since one theme of this book is neuroimaging, it is appropriate to make a few remarks regarding the early compression of the ventricle ipsilateral to the contusion due to edema and its subsequent enduring enlargement. The early compression is usually

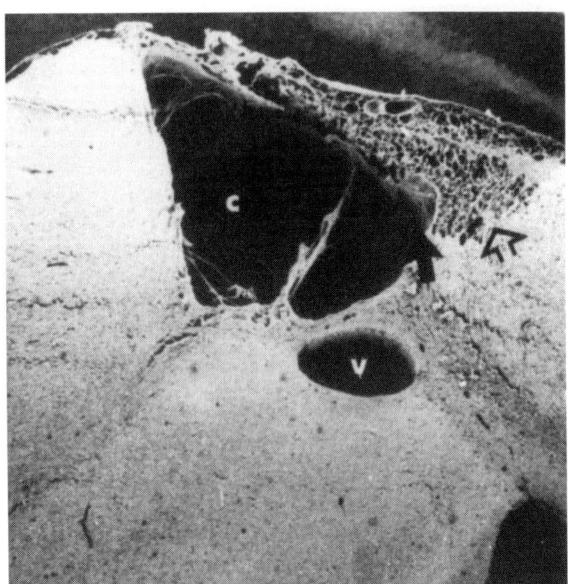

Figure 11-5. Scanning electron microscopic illustrating the final stage in the evolution of a contusion into a fluid-filled cavity. This injury was produced by a 200 gm/cm injury and is 15 days after injury (c = cavity, v = ventricle). This illustration reveals surviving axonal bridges spanning the cavity, which is compatible with the very slow growth of the cavity. The honeycombed cortex (*arrow*) and axonal bridges seen at two weeks are absent one month after injury, likely engulfed by cytotoxic processes. (*Photograph courtesy of H. Murray; manuscript in preparation.*)

associated with a midline shift and expansion of the ipsilateral hemisphere. The enlargement is frequently dismissed as the *ex vacuo* ventricular expansion into vacated space. Also, the behavioral consequences of posttraumatic hydrocephalus are rarely examined in laboratory studies of the effects of experimental lesions. In this TBI model ventricular enlargement is frequently observed weeks after TBI, regardless of extent of cortical necrosis (14). The magnitude of ventricular enlargement after contusion is not correlated with the volume of necrotic cavitation, which excludes the argument that the enlargement is *ex vacuo,* indicating it is posttraumatic hydrocephalus. Ventricular dilation after SMCX ablation is much less than that observed after contusion. Furthermore, the ependymal lining of the ventricles appears disrupted following contusion, but not ablation. Preliminary observations indicate gliosis adjacent to the ependymal breakdown in the enlarged ventricles following TBI, but not ablation injury (14). Since posttraumatic hydrocephalus is an often reported consequence of brain injury in humans (15), this model of TBI would prove useful in delineating the mechanisms of this reaction. To my knowledge, posttraumatic hydrocephalus has not been systematically investigated in other TBI models.

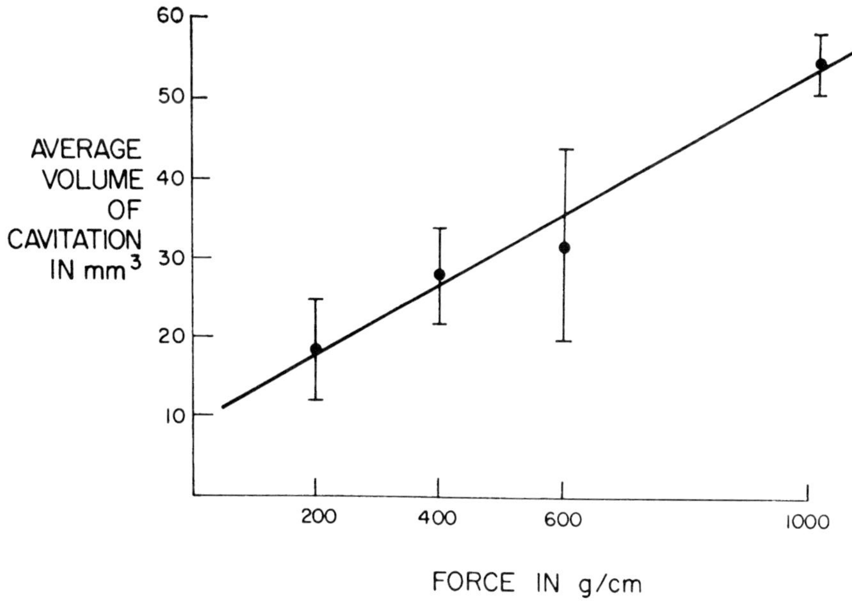

Figure 11-6. Impact trauma dose-response curve for volume of necrotic cavitation measured at 15 days after injury. This data was obtained from animals injured under pentobarbital anesthesia with ketamine given as a preanesthetic. Replication of the 400 gm/cm injury under halothane anesthesia indicated the cavity volume was within one standard error indicating the reliability of the method despite anesthetic changes. The selective neuronal injury in hippocampus illustrated in Figure 11-8 is attenuated by ketamine pretreatment (16,17) but not the extent of cortical injury and thalamic degeneration. This suggests that different pathological processes are involved in these two types of injuries. The severity of the initial symptoms is correlated with the impact force but the rate of recovery from the initial deficit is unaffected. (*Reproduced from Feeney et al., 1981, with permission.*)

Hippocampal Selective Neuronal Injury After TBI

The marked hippocampal subcortical SNI after focal cortical trauma (16,17,18,19) must produce different symptoms than the cortical injury and may result from posttraumatic seizure activity. To determine which of the behavioral deficits following TBI is related to which of the many pathological reactions after this injury is a major problem. As a beginning, it is essential to compare TBI-induced injury to that following selected injury to structures affected by TBI. Similar hippocampal neuronal death can be produced by electrical stimulation inducing hippocampal epileptiform activity (20,21). The SNI in hippocampus, medial geniculate, and dorsolateral caudate does not follow SMCX suction ablation even when using sensitive stains for detecting neuronal death (16,17). Compared to cortical contusion, SNI is subtle, more variable, and was not noted in our first publications describing the injury produced by the weight drop trauma model (4) However, reexamination of the original tissue from those studies showed a reliable pattern of subcortical selective neuronal death, pyramidal neuronal loss in the hippocampal CA3a sector and hilar sectors only in the ipsilateral hemisphere (17). A similar pattern of SNI has been described by others using fluid percussion TBI model (18,19). In contrast to the slow neuronal death at the site of contusion noted previously, hippocampal SNI is completed quite rapidly. By six hours after impact CA3 pyramidal and hilar neurons lose their affinity for Nissl stains and are acidophilic and argyrophilic, indicated by acid fuschin and Fink-Heimer staining. After 400 g/cm weight drop injury to SMCX, SNI is only in the hemisphere ipsilateral to the trauma and the hippocampal reaction is illustrated in Figure 11-7. The CA3 neuronal death, without notable CA1 loss, is unique to TBI and hilar neurons are sensitive to many insults. After fluid percussion, hippocampal SNI can be bilateral or unilateral, and whether the CA3 or hilar neuronal death is greater depends on unknown variables (18,19).

The cause of the distant cell loss is not known but there are several possibilities. One of particular relevance is the excessive release of excitatory amino acid neurotransmitters, especially glutamate and aspartate. In the hippocampal system, Sloviter (20) and others (21) have shown that excessive and sustained activation of entorhinal inputs to dentate gyrus can produce a loss of somatostatin-positive hilar neurons. Sloviter reported that the hippocampal injury is unilateral or bilateral depending on whether the stimulation induced epileptiform activity is unilateral or bilateral (20). We have recorded epileptiform unit activity persisting almost continuously for up to three hours in the ipsi- but not the contralateral hippocampus in weight drop contused rats (22). The single unit activity of CA3 neurons after contusion alternated between bursts of high frequency (maximum of 1000 Hz), long duration (as long as 3.5 min) discharge and periods of quiescence with large field potentials of unknown origin. This alternating pattern usually subsided after three hours and was confined to the hippocampus ipsilateral to the injury. During this time the CA3 region of the contralateral hippocampus showed episodes of complete absence of spontaneous unit activity, presumably due to commissural evoked inhibition. The contralateral hippocampal neurons returned to baseline patterns of activity by three hours after TBI. At twenty-four hours after injury, few neurons could be found in the CA3 region of the ipsilateral hippocampus and the contralateral hippocampus was quite normal.

Others have recorded generalized seizure activity followed by postictal depression in most rats within minutes after a very mild weight drop impact injury (23). In all rats contused under halothane anesthesia and videotaped for careful observation, at least one generalized tonic/clonic convulsion is seen in the first few hours after discontinuing anesthesia (12). Persistent unilateral epileptiform activity may give rise to SNI in some vulnerable structures such as CA3 and hilar regions. However, the mechanism of SNI following TBI or hypoxia/ischemia is uncertain. Both hilar cell loss and hippocampal pyramidal cell loss have been described after unilateral SMCX contusion reportedly without convulsions (19). However, the EEG was not recorded, nor were the animals videotaped for careful study. The authors argued that the cause of the hippocampal cell loss cannot be attributable to seizures since the rats were anesthetized with barbiturate, which blocks generalized convulsions. However, barbiturate only attenuates and does not block interictal activity, the high frequency neuronal activity similar to the stimulation that can produce neuronal injury in CA3 (20,21). In experimental temporal lobe

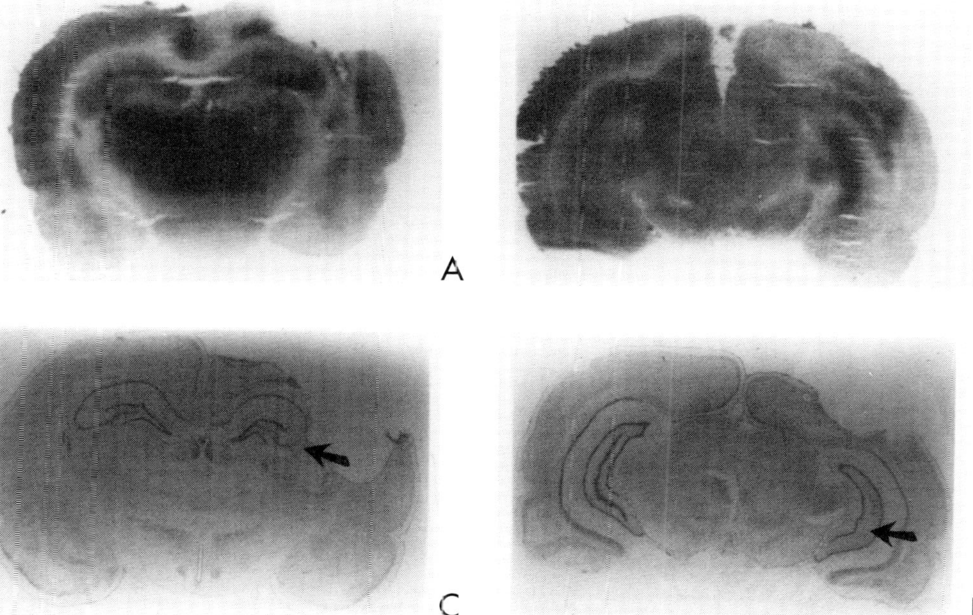

Figure 11-7. Illustrations of remote functional disturbances and selective neuronal injury by the 2 deoxyglucose autoradiography method (A & B, 4 days post) and comparable thionin stained sections (C & D, 30 days post). Tissue processed from animals after a 400 gm/cm injury. (A) Autoradiogram illustrating glucose utilization from a section through the center of the impact. Note the hypermetabolism in the ipsilateral hippocampus especially the CA3 region and cortex adjacent to the injury. (B) Autoradiogram from a section taken posterior to the impact shows high glucose utilization in the ipsilateral ventral hippocampus and CA3 region. Cortex just posterior to the impact is markedly hypometabolic whereas adjacent lateral cortex shows a marked increase in glucose metabolism. In contrast to these transient effects the ipsilateral temporal parietal cortex and amygdala remained hypometabolic for the 16 day duration of the study. (C) Thionin stained section showing loss of CA3a pyramidal neurons (*arrow*) and thalamic gliosis. (D) Thionin stained section illustrating loss of ventral hippocamapal CA3 neurons and gliosis (*arrow*). (*Data from Chen et al., 1988, reproduced with permission.*)

focal epilepsy in cats, moderate interictal activity has been reported to markedly disrupt behavior (24) and so epileptiform after discharge or seizures may not be required for functional and anatomical disturbances. After brain injury in human beings producing contusions with enduring symptoms, as in these TBI models, the percentage of cases developing posttraumatic epilepsy exceeds 60% (25).

Remote Functional Depression (Diaschisis)

It has been proposed that some symptoms of brain injury result from a remote functional depression (RFD), a concept recently formulated to replace the older theory of diaschisis diagrammed in Figure 11-8 (26,27). RFD can be manifest as depressed (or excessive) neuronal metabolism (see Figure 11-7 and Figure 11-9), or some other neuronal perturbation such as altered transmitter release (see Figure 11-12) in morphologically intact structures. The concept has important scientific and clinical implications. If RFD contributes to symptoms, our maps of localization of function, based on only a description of the primary lesion, are misleading. Second, most research on experimental treatments for TBI have utilized anatomical measures of the areas of neuronal death to

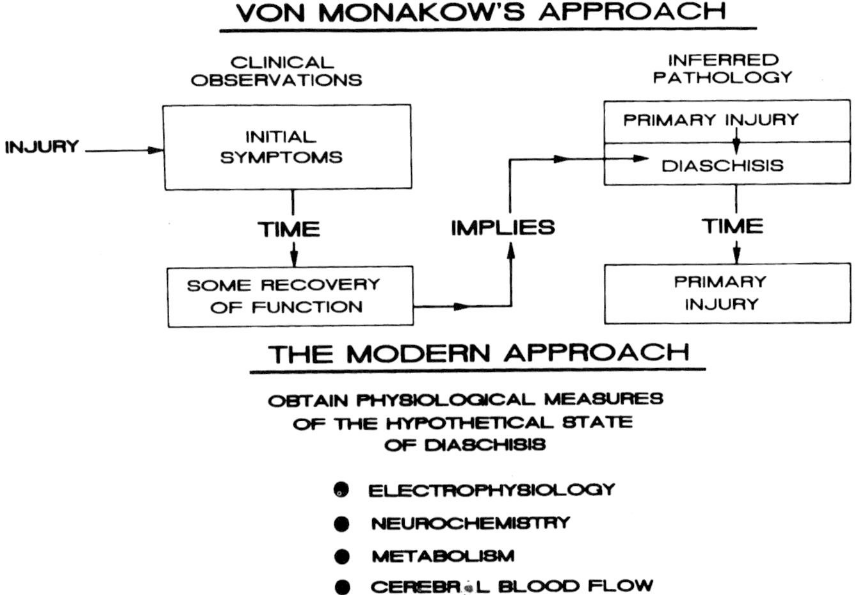

Figure 11-8. Diagram of von Monakow's inference of diaschisis and current measurement techniques. The central problem with von Monakow's approach was that the concept had a circular definition. Since the functional disturbances thought to be the basis of diaschisis could not be measured in that era, the concept was nothing more than another name, with untested assumptions, for recovery of function. The Modern Approach refers to the measurement of functional disturbances in morphologically intact tissue remote from the locus of the injury. *(Feeney, J Neuro Rehab, 1991, reproduced with permission.)*

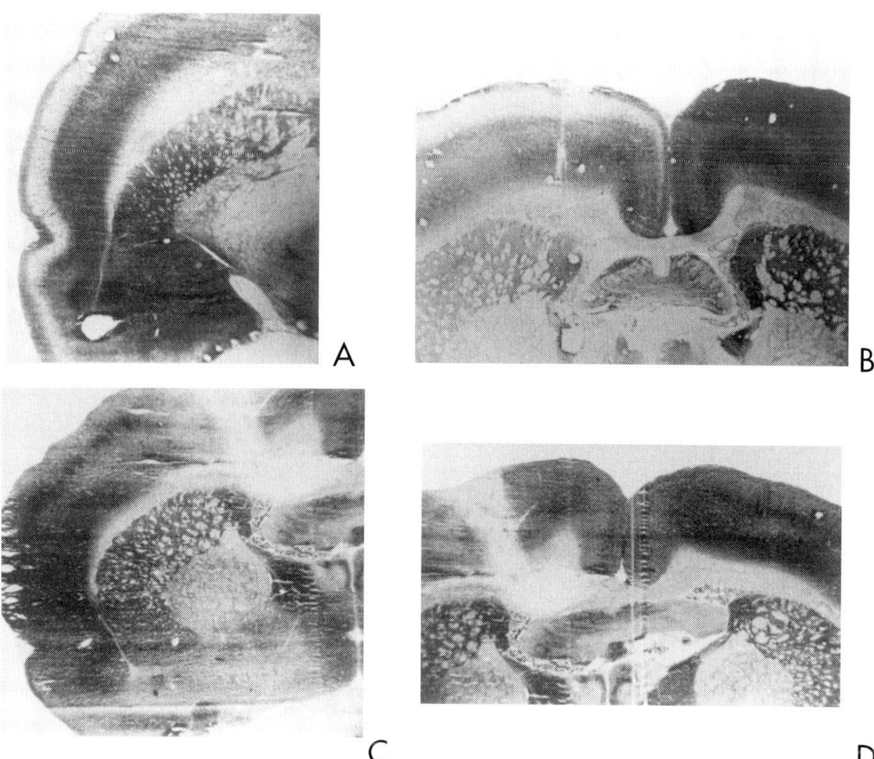

Figure 11–9. Sections stained for the glycolytic enzyme α-glycerophosphate dehydrogenase (α-GPDH) four days following a unilateral SMCX injury. Lack of stain indicates a widespread reduced glycolytic metabolism remote from the injury throughout the ipsilateral cortex. The pale band in the cortex in A indicates that cortical layers 2 and 3 have the most severe depletion of this enzyme in most if the injured hemisphere, extending into temporal neocortex. As illustrated in B. Only some medial cortex is spared the α-GPDH depletion. C and D are also sections taken 4 days after SMCX injury from rats given a single low dose of d-amphetamine 24 hours after injury. The α-GPDH depletion is blocked by the same treatment that promotes functional recovery. (*Feeney, J Neuro Rehab, 1991, reproduced with permission.*)

assess treatment effects. Using only that approach, experimental treatment effects on symptoms resulting from neuronal dysfunction would be overlooked. The increased use of measures of cerebral metabolism in studies of treatments and mechanisms of the symptoms of brain injury (26) will overcome this bias.

It is widely accepted that some types of selective neuronal *death* distant from an infarct or TBI site can be a result of "excitotoxicity" (28,29); the more common neuronal *injury* has received less attention. To account for neuronal dysfunction after brain injury, I proposed that excessive but sublethal EAA receptor activation may be the cellular mechanism leading to RFD (27). According to this "soft excitotoxicity hypothesis," focal brain injury results in widespread metabolic depression from the disruption of ionic homeostasis in neurons injured, but not killed, by exposure to the massive amounts of EAAs. Abnormally high glutamate and aspartate release has been detected in areas remote from an infarct or contusion using microdialysis (23,30). These areas of high EAA release without evidence of neuronal injury show some characteristics of RFD, or diaschisis (26,27), reduced CBF, and energy depletion (30). It has been suggested that the absence of neuronal death in these regions is due to an abundance of inhibitory transmitters, GABA and glycine. Thus a regional imbalance between excitation and inhibition has been proposed to account for selective vulnerability after brain injury (31). The massive EAA release in the first minutes following TBI has been reported to be highly correlated with generalized seizure activity (23) and if recurring as in our model (12,22) could produce neuronal metabolic disturbances . We have reported hypo- and hypermetabolism revealed by autoradiograhic measures of glucose utilization (see Figure 11-7) (32). We reported similar results after TBI and motor cortex ablation in rat and cat for oxidative metabolism revealed by the histochemical stain for the mitochondrial enzyme cytochrome oxidase (32,33).

Metabolic disturbances after TBI are much more complex than morphological injury. Nevertheless, some progress has been made in clinical studies of the mechanisms and behavioral correlates of metabolic perturbations remote from a focal brain injury. In clinical studies, different results are obtained dependent upon the techniques used to measure metabolism (34), the time after brain damage (36), or the behavior of the patient while being tested (36). Similarly, complexities are reported in laboratory studies. For example, depending on the method used to measure glycolytic metabolism, different patterns of disturbances following TBI have been described. Using the histochemical stain for the glycolytic enzyme α-glycerophosphate dehydrogenase (α-GPDH), we described a marked depletion of the enzyme (37). This occurs throughout most of the cortex ipsilateral to focal brain injury and persists for as long as nine days (see Figure 11-9). This effect on a measure of glucose metabolic capacity is quite different from that measured for glucose utilization. The pattern of α-GPDH reduction, not affecting part of the medial cortex and most prominent in cortical layers II and III, as illustrated in Figure 11-9, is similar to the reported increase in glucose utilization after a single epoch of spreading depression but was originally considered unrelated (37). However, reconsideration of the data suggested this slow developing, enduring, and robust depletion of a glycolytic enzyme in almost the entire cortical mantle ipsilateral to the injury was attributable to repeated episodes of spreading depression (27). This hypothesis has only recently received experimental support and so deserves some discussion. Lee et al. (38) recently reported that large waves of depolarization, similar to spreading depression, appear for several hours following cortical contusions. Since spreading depression is a neuronal dysfunction, it would be included in the concepts of RFD or diaschisis (26,27). Depletion of the glycolytic enzyme in the cortex may reflect lowered neuronal activity. This reduction of a glycolytic enzyme in the cortex of the injured hemisphere of the rat may be related to alterations in CBF in stroke patients. A minor (19%) but extensive and enduring reduction of CBF over the "periinfarct area," extending to over 30% of the injured hemisphere, has been reported after stroke (39). The behavioral consequences, if any, of this metabolic disturbance after TBI are unknown.

Measures of Symptoms of Functional Outcome

Locomotor Deficits

To measure the hemiplegia in rat after SMCX trauma, I designed a beam walking task and a performance rating scale to measure recovery from hemiplegia (40). The training/adaptation of the rat to the testing procedure only takes a few days and has been described in detail elsewhere (12,13). Testing requires only a few minutes per animal every other day for two weeks. Unlike running speed or the rotorod test (discussed below), the rating scale measures whether the animal can traverse the beam and, most importantly, how it uses the affected limbs. On this scale, animals are scored "1" if unable to maintain their balance on the beam, "2" if unable to traverse the beam, but placed their affected limbs on the surface of the beam at least once and maintained their balance on the beam. As illustrated in Figure 11-10, by five to seven days after a 400g/cm injury, the rats will score "5," indicating they traversed the beam and used their affected limbs in fewer than half their steps along the beam. They subsequently recover to the normal, preinjury baseline score of "7."

Using this task, the rats appear to "recover" quickly, returning to baseline beam walk test performance within two weeks after injury. However, these rats are not fully recovered. If the task is made more demanding or by pharmacological challenge with drugs blocking (1 NA transmission discussed below and elsewhere in detail (13,27), deficits can be "reinstated" in injured animals. These observations indicate that for some period after apparent recovery the CNS is maintaining function of locomotor circuitry at a limited capacity that can be "unmasked" by α_1 noradrenergic receptor challenged.

We have also used this task, with a slightly modified rating scale, in the cat to measure hemiplegia recovery after unilateral (41) or bilateral frontal cortex ablation (42). The cat is very disabled for a prolonged period, at least a few months, depending on the extent of the lesion, and the symptoms are striking. Some symptoms are permanent; for example, there is a permanent loss of tactile placing reflexes (43) lasting for as long as seven years (Feeney, unpublished observations). The beam walk outcome measure is very useful for evaluating drug effects on recovery after experimental brain injury (13) since it is inexpensive, easy to implement, and behavioral testing is completed within two weeks. Moreover, it is readily adaptable to other species, and data based on this outcome evaluation of drug effects have been extended to patients with brain injury (7,8). Additionally, we often measure forepaw and/or vibrissae reflexes (43,45) and occasionally use the more laborious tests of forepaw grasping deficits in the rat (46), which are thought to reflect the extent and severity of the cortical injury. This use of multiple measures has proven useful since although they are all consequences of TBI, as discussed below, they respond to different treatments. We have compared the seemingly crude locomotor rating scale measurement to more apparently quantitative measurements such as running speed, gait analysis using pawprint measurements, and more complex devices to study locomotor agility. There is a slowing of running speed after SMCX injury in the rat (47), which some investigators use as a dependent variable on the beam walk task. But there are limitations with this measure. After a few days injured animals may run the length of the beam as quickly as the control uninjured group but with obvious hemiplegic symptoms, so running speed measurement omits potentially important, easily gathered data. Additionally, running speed is markedly affected by motivational factors (48) that do not bias the rating scale measure of locomotor ability. Some years ago, we evaluated the rotorod test, which measures the time duration rats stay on a rotating drum as a measure of hemiplegia recovery after SMCX injury in rat (Feeney, unpublished observations). This test is commonly used in toxicology as an index of CNS pathology. The major shortcoming with this method is that one has no idea why the animal falls from the rotorod device. While such crude descriptions of CNS pathology are adequate for detecting toxicity, for TBI one would prefer to have some understanding of the symptoms under study or being treated. Unlike the recent report (49) describing the rotorod test as useful for assessment of functional recovery following fluid percussion injury, we found it much less sensitive than the rating scale after impact contusion. This difference in sensitivity of measures is evidently dependent upon the model employed. Sutton (personal communication) has replicated both our findings in contusion and the different results using the fluid percussion model. This may indicate important differences in the injuries produced by impact trauma and fluid percussion. Most recently we attempted to analyze recovery from hemiplegia by measuring pawprint patterns to analyze disturbances in gait. To our surprise, the very labor-intensive pawprint measures to assess gait in the hemiplegic rat were not as sensitive a measure of hemiplegia recovery as beam walk assessment. However it is useful for differentiating injury to systems that appear similar using the beam walk rating scale (50).

Postural Alterations

Examination of motor and postural disturbances after TBI or ablation of the SMCX in rat or cat indicates much more complex symptomatology than summarized in the beam walk score. The symptoms include many components of hemiplegia observed in human beings. Pathological grasp can be readily observed in rat (51) and cat under the correct conditions, and the abnormal posture is most striking in the cat after unilateral frontal cortex ablation. Early after injury when in the quadruped position, rats and especially cats display forelimb extension and splaying of the digits. In contrast, when the animals are arched into a bipedal position, the affected forepaw flexes, the digits clench, and the affected hindlimb extends. Hemiplegic patients reportedly show arm extension when placed in a quadruped position (Professor A. Earl Walker, personal communication). The reversal of abnormal posture following sensorimotor cortex injury by changing body position suggests it is under vestibular control. The locomotor deficits and postural disturbances after injury to the cerebral cortex are hypothesized to result from cerebellar dysfunction.

Learning and Memory Deficits

Both rats and human beings have enduring learning and memory deficits after brain injury, and this extensive topic has been discussed in detail by others (52). Memory deficits in the rat after hippocampal injury are often measured using the Morris maze, which requires learning and memory of the spatial arrangement of cues for the animal to efficiently escape from a pool (53). After TBI in the rat there is a loss of spatial learning ability measured using the Morris maze (18,19,54–56). In the weight drop model, the data from studies using the standard Morris water task indicate an enduring, selective learning impairment, not a global "cognitive" deficit of all complex task problem solving. At one hundred days posttrauma, when tested in the maze with a visible escape platform, neither learning ability nor swim speeds of the injured rats were different from controls. The apparently normal performance on this task excludes interpretation of Morris maze deficits after TBI as due to motivational, sensory, or motor problems. However, if the platform were hidden, requiring spatial navigation using a more complex, indirect set of cues from the test room, injured rats showed a learning deficit. With practice, however, they could eventually perform as well as control animals. Moreover, when the platform was removed the rats with TBI went to the correct quadrant as frequently as normal rats. This indicates that they know the location of the escape platform but are slower to learn or utilize spatial cues. Together these data suggest that TBI produces a unilateral hippocampal CA3 and hilar sector injury accompanied by a permanent spatial learning impairment different from that after large bilateral hippocampal neurotoxin lesions (55). Additionally, after TBI but not SMCX ablation, electrophysiological measures of field potentials indicate a normal hippocampal input/output response curve but a selective loss of LTP in the hippocampus ipsi- but not contralateral to the injury (56). Enduring learning and memory impairment only follows bilateral hippocampal destruction (52). Either there is something unique about the hippocampal damage produced by TBI or unilateral hippocampal injury together with the other brain damage produced by TBI produces this enduring spatial learning impairment.

Experimental Pharmacological Treatment of Contusions and SNI

The differing neuropathologies and symptoms produced by the weight drop injury undoubtedly are multiply determined, produced by diverse events such as excitotoxicity, acidosis, ischemia, and free radical formation. For any particular pathology, one process may predominate and its impact may be lessened by pharmacological blockade. This logic has only proven to be of limited success. In this section only excitotoxicity and acidosis are discussed, and ischemia is briefly mentioned. There have been recent comprehensive reviews of pharmacological treatments for brain injury (58,59), and data from pharmacological screening studies in this TBI model were recently summarized (60). Therefore, I will briefly describe the putative mechanisms and mention only a few representative drug studies for each of the three pathological reactions that are the theme of this chapter.

Excitotoxicity

Some drugs are considered to exert neuroprotection by interference with excitotoxicity involving the N-methyl-D-aspartate (NMDA) EAA receptor complex subtype. The NMDA receptor has been well-studied with selective antagonists, such as ketamine and MK-801. The non-NMDA subclasses of EAA receptors, kainate and quisqualate (28,29), may mediate similar cellular events, perhaps characteristic of voltage sensitive Ca2+ ion channels. The NMDA channel, when excessively activated, can produce delayed cell death (completed within a few days) from extreme disturbances of ionic conduction and homeostasis resulting in diverse intracellular pathology (29). Excitotoxicity can be attenuated by NMDA antagonists (29) but additional studies of functional benefit are required. There is pharmacological evidence that the NMDA receptor predominantly mediates the SNI in hippocampus but not the pancellular necrosis. We found that pre- or post-TBI treatment (5 minutes) with ketamine, a selective NMDA noncompetitive antagonist, reduced the extent of hippocampal CA3 pyramidal cell loss. However, this treatment had no detectable effect on the extent of cortical injury, nor did it improve beam walk recovery (16,17). Interpretation of the mechanism of such results must be cautious. Even for such a well-studied compound as the noncompetitive NMDA receptor antagonist MK-801, there are data to support the alternative hypothesis that its *in vivo* neuroprotection is attributable to effects on CBF (61). Additionally, the "rescue" of neurons does not necessarily translate into improved function. The decreased neuronal death in the substania nigra by pharmacological intervention has been reported to worsen symptoms (62). Ketamine also markedly lowers body temperature, a procedure known to be neuroprotective (63), and temperature has not always been controlled in studies of its neuroprotective action.

Acidosis

A qualitatively different pharmacological approach to neuroprotection is to reduce acidosis. Moreover, pannecrosis is usually attributed to acidosis (64). There is documentation that in some hypoxia/ischemia models, insulin administration at the time of insult has neuroprotective effects on both extent of injury and functional outcome. Conversely, there are both experimental and clinical data reporting that hyperglycemia worsens ischemic brain damage (64–67); however, the mechanisms underlying these effects are less clear than those of NMDA antagonists. Some attribute the beneficial effects to increasing the depressed metabolic capacity of injured neurons, enhancing their ability to maintain ionic homeostasis and/or reduction of lactate acidosis (68). Glucose starvation or other metabolic perturbations of cerebellar granule cells leads to sufficient depolarization to relieve the Mg++ block of the NMDA channel. This permits low sublethal doses of glutamate to cause a rapid influx of both Na+ and Ca++ and if excessive can result in extensive neuronal death (68). Neurons are quite vulnerable in this energy-deprived condition when ion pumps are unable to maintain intracellular homeostasis. There is evidence that following cerebral trauma there is a short duration NMDA mediated hypermetabolic state (69), which can be blocked by antagonists. During this condition of energy depletion neuronal capacity to regulate excessive ionic influx due to elevated EAA exposure would be compromised. A reduced energy state may weaken cellular responses to post-injury acidosis (70). There are studies indicating an interaction between these mechanisms leading to cell death. Exposure of neurons to glutamate produces a prolonged intracellular decrease in pH as a result of increased H ion concentration. At two or more hours following exposure to toxic levels of glutamate, the H ion concentration did not return and stabilize at baseline levels, but progressively increased. Thus, a prolonged acidosis produced by intraneuronal H ion concentration increase could act synergistically with calcium ion influx to produce secondary neuronal injury (70). We have reported (45) and recently replicated an experimental observation that posttraumatic insulin administration promotes recovery of tactile placing in the rat without affecting beam walk recovery. For reasons mentioned previously, vestibular modifications of hemiplegic posture, and data presented below we hypothesized that hemiplegia after SMCX injury results from cerebellar dysfunction (28) and did not predict an effect of insulin on this symptom. In our first insulin study we found no reduction of the volume of the necrotic cavitation but will conduct more precise reconstruction of the cortical injury from histology of our recent replication of the insulin effect on recovery of tactile placing. The effects of blood glucose manipulations on secondary neuronal injury have been reviewed without simple conclusions and indicate the necessity to examine different "types" of secondary neuronal injury or different effects in different regions (71).

Noradrenergic Modulation of Remote Functional Depression

Interest in a potential pharmacotherapy for brain injury was first formally reported shortly after identification of the neurotransmitter acetylcholine. To investigate effects on recovery of function, studies manipulating every known or putative neurotransmitter have been conducted [for a review of the early era of pharmacological studies of recovery of functions, see (46)]. After years of disappointing clinical results, interest resumed in the 1980s. The renewed interest was based on several developments, including extensive research characterizing the physiological events initiated by injury and several experimental observations. Pharmacological NMDA receptor blockade in the first hours after brain injury, as described previously, could rescue neurons destined for death following TBI, due to "excitotoxicity." However, the clinical utility of this approach has not been validated (61) and may be quite limited because of the necessity for intervention within the first few hours after injury. Perhaps the most important aspect of the experimental treatment to be discussed is that it is effective even when initiated weeks after cortical injury.

The study of effects of amphetamine on recovery of function has a long history [see (46)]. It was resurrected by our report (40) that a single administration of a low dose of amphetamine, even when given one day after unilateral SMCX TBI or ablation, accelerated recovery from hemiplegia in rat. This effect after moderate but not severe TBI is illustrated in Figure 11-10. To achieve this result with a single dose, it was necessary to provide symptom relevant experience (SRE; i.e., physical therapy) during the period of drug action. This intervention is not a panacea, lacking effects on forepaw grasping in the same animals showing facilitated recovery of locomotor deficits (see Figure 11-11). We then described a similar enhancement of recovery from hemiplegia in the cat, also measured by beam walk testing. Importantly, this effect was dramatic even though treatment was not initiated until ten days after unilateral

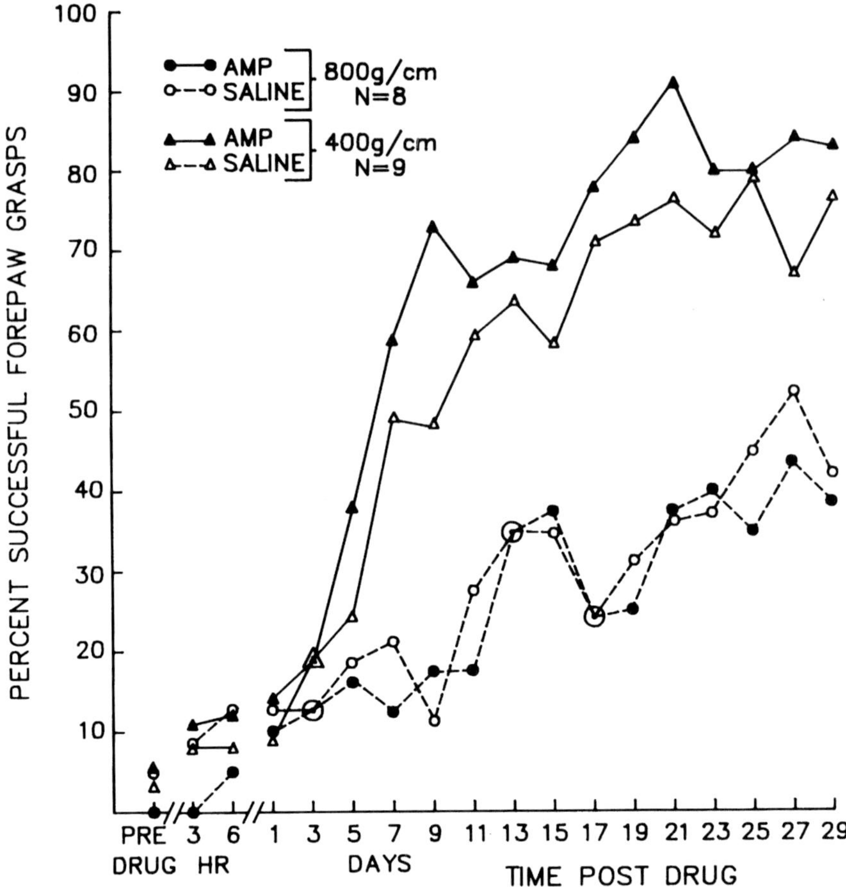

Figure 11-10. Enhancement of recovery from hemipegia by a single administration of a low dose of amphetamine following moderate, but not severe, SMCX contusion. Mean ratings of rat beam walk test ability after unilateral injury (400 or 800 gm/cm) to the right SMCX. Animals with a 400 gm/cm contusion were administered 2 mg/kg of d-amphetamine or saline 24 hours after injury immediately following the pre drug test. A significant enhancement of beam walk ability was observed on the first test one hour post drug and facilitated recovery remained significant for 3 days following treatment. Subsequent replications suggest that a higher dosage is optimal in trauama and embolic stroke models than after SMCX ablation. Animals with the 800 gm/cm did not show any improved beam walk ability even when administered a second treatment on day 3 posttrauma. (*Reproduced from Feeney and Sutton, 1988, with permission.*)

frontal cortex ablation. As in the rat, enhanced recovery required SRE and was not a transient drug effect but endured long after the drug had been metabolized. On the beam walk task using the rating scale modified for the cat, treated animals were fully recovered by twenty-one days after injury and maintained the recovery from

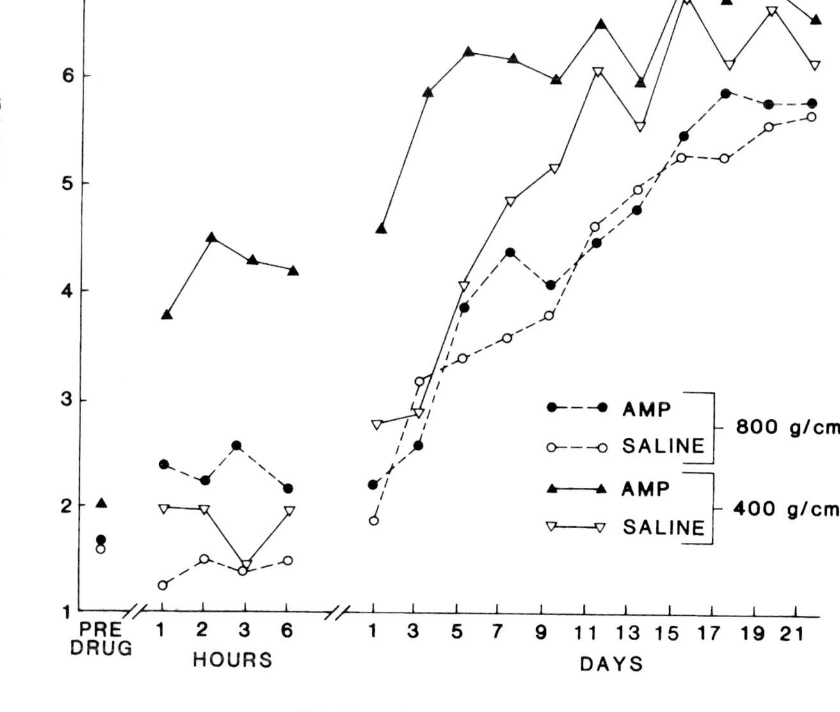

Figure 11-11. Recovery of forepaw grasping from the same rats described in Figure 11-10 was unaffected by amphetamine treatment. Grasping ability was measured by percent retrieval of food pellets using the left forepaw after right SMCX contusion. (*Reproduced from Feeney and Sutton, 1988, with permission.*)

hemiplegia. Untreated control cats did not recover in the sixty days of the experiment. This treatment was even more dramatic in cats with large bilateral frontal ablations (44), which excluded any role of homotypical cortex in hemiplegia recovery. These severely disabled cats required three treatments spaced at four-day intervals to achieve recovery, whereas the control group showed little improvement. This multiple treatment regimen and scheduling drug administration with an interval of several days avoided the complicating effects of chronic administration and served as a model paradigm for clinical studies (7,8).

To test this treatment on the symptoms of an experimental stroke, we developed a rat embolic stroke model not requiring anesthesia during the infarct nor any violation of the cranium (72). Emboli were made by fragmenting homologous blood clots and were injected into a catheter that had been previously implanted into one carotid artery after tying off the external carotid, which innervates the rat face. These emboli primarily occlude end arterioles of one middle cerebral artery and produce the symptoms of acute stroke, a severe and enduring hemiplegia, seizures, and weight loss. This model is useful for testing a potential therapy, but because of the high mortality rate and difficult surgery it is not useful for drug screening. Fifty percent of saline treated rats died within the first week after infusion of emboli. Surprisingly, no treated rats died, an unexpected significant mortality reduction. This would not have been detected using a typical drug screening model of recovery of function. The severe locomotor deficit was not improved by a single administration but was alleviated by multiple administrations or short-term, very low dose continuous infusion by osmotic minipump for seven days. This infusion produced no anorexia in normal rats and, paradoxically, treated stroke rats lost less body weight than saline controls. Moreover, when treated, severely disabled stroke rats recovered locomotor agility to baseline levels while control animals still had severe locomotor disabilities thirty days post-infarct (72). The applicability of this NE/SRE approach to the treatment of stroke symptoms in human beings has been recently reviewed (7,8).

There is now considerable evidence supporting the idea that the beneficial effects of amphetamine on recovery from hemiplegia as mediated by increased activity at central α_1 NA receptors. As reviewed elsewhere (13,58,60), all drugs tested that directly or indirectly increase activity at α_1 NA synapses improve recovery. The family of drugs tested, which have the same effect on functional recovery as amphetamine, range from the over-the-counter drug phenolpropanolamine (73) to the synthetic NE precursor, L-DOPS, which increases NE release and levels. Importantly, the same investigators also evaluated L-DOPS for therapeutic effects in a diverse population of hemiplegic stroke patients using the same measure as in the other clinical studies (74). The drug significantly enhanced functional recovery even when treatment was initiated one month after the stroke. This rapid testing of a laboratory effect in a patient population was possible because of the extensive clinical experience with L-DOPS in Japan, where it is often used to treat some of the late stages of Parkinsonism. These studies exclude interpretation of this "amphetamine effect" as due to stimulant properties that are absent after administration of L-DOPS. The antidepressant desipramine, like L-DOPS, lacks stimulant properties but blocks NE reuptake. This antidepressant also facilitates recovery from hemiplegia in the rat ablation model (75).

If interpretation of the mechanism of this effect is correct and increased α_1 NA activity improves recovery from hemiplegia, then drugs reducing activity at these synapses should slow recovery. This hypothesis has received strong support from laboratory and clinical studies. Drugs that reduce α_1 NA activity slow hemiplegia recovery and also dramatically reinstate symptoms long after SMCX ablation (at least one month in rat, and after years in the cat). This transient effect persists for several hours in apparently recovered animals at a dose having no effect on beam walk performance in sham operate controls. The α_1 NA antagonists, prazosin and phenoxybenzamine, slow recovery and reinstate deficits in both SMCX contused or ablated animals following complete recovery of beam-walking ability. The reinstatement is not due to a nonspecific soporific drug effect since the deficits reappear only in the limbs contralateral to the injury and do not appear after a sedating dose of pentobarbital (76–79). Increased activity at α_2 NA autoreceptors reduce NE release at α_1 NA synapses because of negative feedback action on locus coeruleus somata and terminals. The theoretical prediction that α_2 NA agonists will slow recovery and reinstate hemiplegic symptoms has also been supported. The commonly prescribed antihypertensive clonidine, an α_2 NA agonist, retards hemiplegia recovery after SMCX ablation in the rat (80,81). Conversely, the highly selective α_2 NA agonist, idazoxane, promotes hemiplegia recovery (82). Since the β NA agonist propranolol (60) had no effect on recovery in the hemiplegic rat model, the set of pharmacological data is consistent with interpretation of the mechanism of drug action via NE acting at α_1 NA receptors.

To directly ascertain if NE mediated these drug effects on recovery from hemiplegia, dose-response studies of intraventricular infusions of monoamine transmitters were compared for effects on beam walk test recovery after SMCX ablation. The results showed that the infusion of NE, but not DA or 5-HT, mimicked the effects of amphetamine on hemiplegia recovery [(83) and unpublished 5-HT data of Feeney, Navratil, and Boyeson]. Additionally, implanting an "endogenous catecholamine minipump" into the wound cavity produced enduring alleviation of some persistent reflex deficits in the cat. This was accomplished by autografting adrenal medulla chromaffin cells into the wound cavity twenty-one days after a large unilateral frontal ablation. Compared to controls or "early grafts" (twelve-day interval) late autografts produced a long-term partial restoration of the contralateral tactile placing response. Tactile placing reflexes were completely absent in the affected limb of untreated cats or early grafted animals for almost one year of the study (60,84). Presumably the graft continues to secrete NE into the CSF analogous to intraventricular infusion and numerous surviving grafts were found in only the "late graft" animals. The intraventricular data combined with the numerous pharmacological studies answered the question of which neurotransmitter was important for promoting functional recovery late after cortical injury. But where that neurotransmitter exerted its beneficial actions remains unclear.

NE Activity in the Cerebellum Modifies Recovery from Hemiplegia

Several lines of evidence suggested that the cerebellum may mediate the modulatory effect of NE on the dysfunctional neurons producing hemiplegia. First, our original hypothesis that the extrapyramidal system, the transmitter dopamine, and the striatum were involved was excluded by experimental data. Apomorphine, a dopaminergic agonist, had no effect in the rat ablation hemiplegia paradigm at any dose tested (46,58,60). Second, we could not produce a beam walk deficit by large unilateral lesions in the striatum (42). Third, cerebellar lesions produced marked beam walk deficits and both amphetamine and haloperidol worsened the cerebellar deficits (85). Fourth, the abnormal postures after unilateral SMCX lesion could be markedly altered by changing vestibular input as described previously, an effect usually attributed to cerebellar function.

Boyeson and Krobert directly tested this NE-cerebellar hypothesis of recovery from hemiplegia (86). They reported that infusion of NE into the cerebellar cortex contralateral, but not ipsilateral, to the SMCX injury facilitated beam walk recovery. Complementing these data is their report of reinstatement of hemiplegia by microinfusion of the α_1 NA antagonist phenoxybenzamine into the cerebellar cortex contralateral, but not ipsilateral, to an SMCX ablation. This infusion reinstates deficits in animals recovered from cortical ablation (87) similar to systemic α_1 NA antagonist administration (76,77).

These treatments apparently reverse an important consequence of SMCX injury, disturbance of the release of NE from locus coeruleus terminals. Studies from several laboratories have indicated that following TBI or SMCX ablation there is a significant reduction of NE levels and α_1 NA receptor binding. Following SMCX injury, the levels of NE are reduced in almost every structure examined (89–91). Moreover, administration of the dose of amphetamine that improves functional recovery also increases NE levels (89). We directly tested our hypothesis (27,46,58,88) of depressed NE synaptic activity due to axotomy of locus coeruleus neurons from a retrograde cellular reaction due to axotomy of its cortical projections as they traverse the SMCX. Using microdialysis with HPLC in awake, behaving rats, we measured the spontaneous and amphetamine evoked release of NE in cerebellar cortex twenty-four hours after SMCX injury after weight drop trauma. As depicted in Figure 11-12, spontaneous release remained significantly depressed twenty-four hours after SMCX trauma, but there are sufficient NE stores to allow a low dose of amphetamine to increase release by 522–1088%, which slowly returned to the depressed baseline in injured rats over the subsequent five hours (91). However, at one hour after SMCX ablation a complete block of amphetamine evoked NE release was reported (92) even though the entire cerebellum was perfused. These data require two modifications of our original proposal (27,46,58,88). The reduced NE release cannot be due to locus coeruleus axotomy, as this would produce a predominately unilateral reduction of spontaneous NE release. However, as illustrated in Figure 11-12, SMCX injury produces a bilateral reduction of NE release in the cerebellum. While axotomy may play some role, it seems more likely that these neurons are functionally depressed by excessive EAA corticofugal input as discussed previously as "soft excitotoxicity." Additionally, counts of locus coeruleus neurons after SMCX injury indicated no ipsilateral contralateral differences nor a difference between injured and sham operates (Feeney and Bramlett, unpublished observations). The reduction of metabolism in the region of the locus coeruleus is bilateral (32). Additionally, the original prediction of a restoration of NE to normal levels after treatment (27,46,58,88) must be modified since the effect on NE is only transient (91). Despite the reduction in NE release and levels by SMCX injury, there is no compensatory increase in α_1 NA receptors. Instead of an upregulation in response to loss of input, two different laboratories have described a chronic loss of α_1 NA receptor binding (93,94).

The experience (SRE) during the period of drug induced release of NE is an important aspect of this treatment. It was originally proposed (27,46,58,88) that release of the neuromodulator NE "enables" SRE inputs to activate the "performance" circuits also depressed by the injury. The SRE inputs are thought to be both corollary discharges

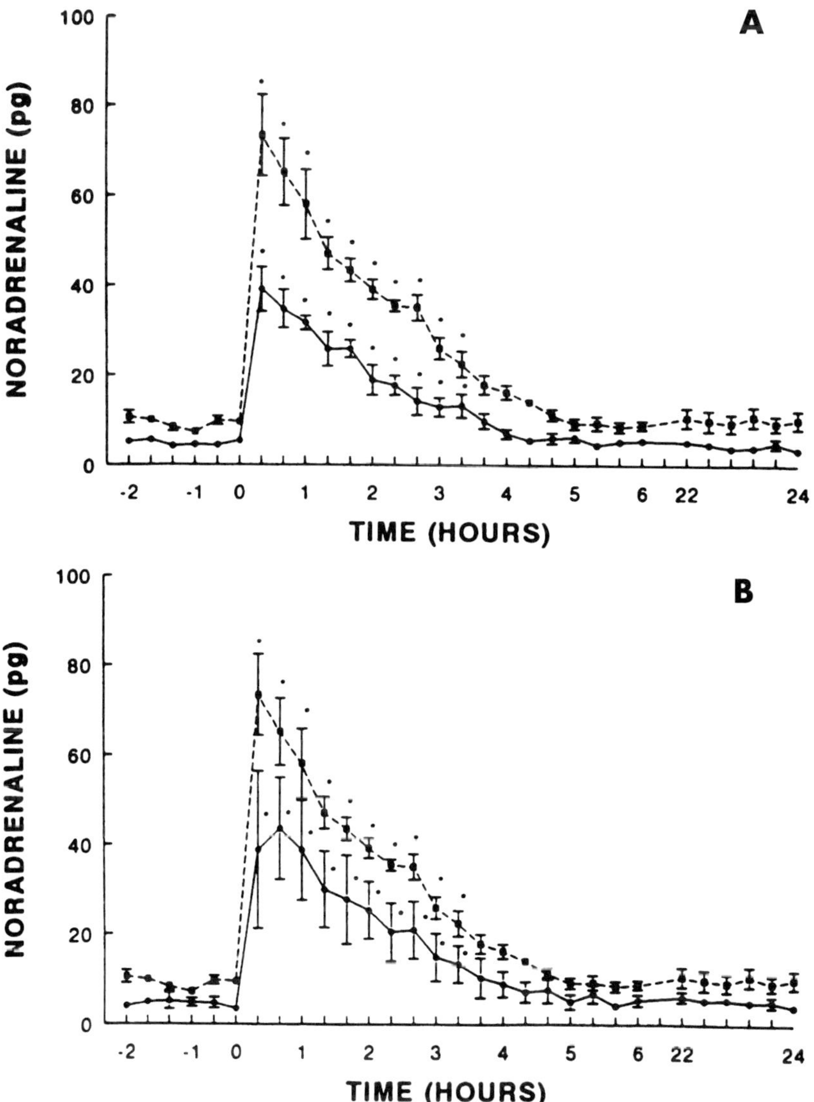

Figure 11-12. Microdialysis measurements showing significantly depressed spontaeous and amphetamine evoked release of noradrenalin (NE) into the extracellular space of the cerebellar cortex 24 hrs after right SMCX contusion. Each data point is the mean (+SEM) amount of NE in 20 minute samples prior to and after amphetamine administration (2mg/kg; ip) taken from the (A) left cerebellar cortex (contralateral to the SMCX injury), or (B) right cerebellar cortex. Solid lines are from rats with SMCX contusion dashed lines are levels from sham operate controls. The difference in spontaneous release prior to drug administration was significant between injured and sham operate controls. Dots above sample points indicate a statistically significant increase above baseline after drug administration. The amphetamine treatment increased NE release for over 3 hours. No significant difference was found between the ipsi- and contralateral cerebellar hemispheres. (*From Krobert et al., 1994, reproduced with permission.*)

from the attempted movement and its proprioceptive feedback (27). These normally interact with such performance circuits to provide corrective adjustments but after injury first interact with NE to alleviate the depressed system. From studies of spontaneous recovery, the red nucleus appears central to the recovery process (50).

NE and Remote Functional Depression (Diaschisis)

It is important to note that the effect of a single dose on a hemiplegic rat or cat with a unilateral cortical injury is immediate. A significant improvement in beam walking is observed on the first beam walk trial thirty minutes after drug administration. This *immediate* effect excluded interpretation of the initial effect as learning, since there was no practice. The enhanced recovery from the treatment was enduring. In the cat the difference between the experimental and control groups remains significant for the sixty days of the experiment. It was this and similar observations (43) that suggested this effect was an alleviation of a diaschisis.

The direct evidence for NE/SRE enhancing functional recovery is supported by parallel studies of drug effects on cerebral metabolism. The areas of reduced glucose utilization, illustrated in Figure 11-7, are normalized by the same treatment that facilitates functional recovery (32). This has also been documented for oxidative metabolism using cytochrome oxidase histochemistry (32,33). Amphetamine alteration of glucose utilization and enhanced behavioral recovery have been reported in the photochemical rat stroke model (95,96). However, the data in that study were considered as evidence for utilization of alternate circuits for recovery. Additionally, the posttraumatic depletion of α-GPDH is blocked by treatment with amphetamine, and locus coeruleus lesions worsen the enzyme depletion (88).

NE and CBF

The mechanisms by which MK-801 and some other drugs are neuroprotective may involve their increasing CBF (61). Since cerebral trauma markedly alters CBF, as does amphetamine, it seemed plausible that it, too, could affect outcome by improving cerebral circulation. Importantly, NE can increase CBF and cerebral metabolism via adrenergic receptors (97). This effect on neuronal metabolism is not necessarily mediated by an effect on CBF since it also occurs in rat cortical tissue slice (97). Interestingly, there are abundant α_1 NA receptors on astrocytes and selective activation of those receptors increases their metabolism (98). A role for glial cells in this effect on neuronal dysfunction is being investigated.

We tested the hypothesis of CBF mediating the amphetamine +SRE effect on hemiplegia recovery after SMCX injury in two experiments. First, we administered a dose of atropine, which blocks the increase of CBF produced by the usual 2 mg/kg dose of amphetamine in rat [see Figure 2 in (58)]. Using this regimen, we still obtained the enduring facilitation of recovery of beam walk performance after SMCX ablation. While this indicates that amphetamine induced increases of CBF are not required for this treatment to improve hemiplegia recovery, it is necessary to directly test the CBF hypothesis. In a second experiment, we used quantitative autoradiographic measurement of rCBF in rats twenty-four hours after cortical contusion dur-

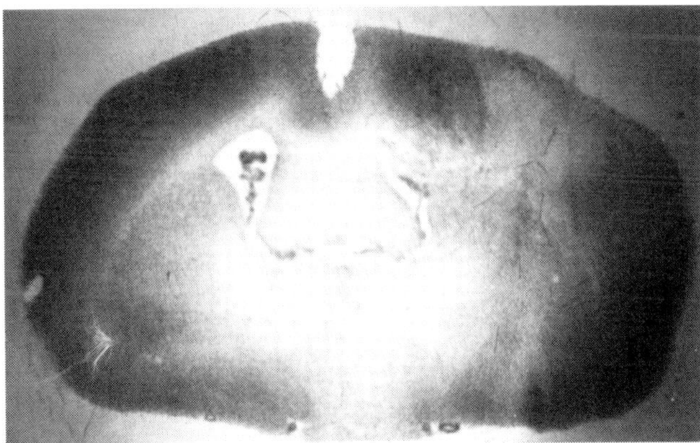

Figure 11-13. An autoradiogram illustrating regional cerebral blood flow (rCBF) at 24 hours after a 400 g/cm SMCX contusion made using C14 iotopyridine. A profound ischemia persists at the site of the impact and a mildly hyperemic area in dosolateral striatum and cortex lateral to the contusion. Although amphetamine (2 mg/kg, ip) bilaterally enhanced CBF, it did not affect the ischemic core or hyperemic areas. The pattern of trauma induced changes in rCBF is not affected by amphetamine indicating the drug's effect on functional recovery is not mediated by improving blood flow in compromised tissue involved in the effect on behavior or metabolism. Also note the compression of the ipsilateral venticle from edema. A pseudocolor version of this illustration is available on the Internet at http://spine.unm.edu/neurogurg/sym/welcome3.html (see Notes Added in Proof). (*Preliminary data from Scremin, O. and Feeney, D.M. Photograph kindly made by M. Wilcox.*)

ing the period of amphetamine action to determine if it normalized perturbed CBF. As illustrated in Figure 11-13, marked changes in regional CBF were observed one day after TBI. An area of severe ischemia was measured in the area that evolves into a contusion, rCBF was 25% of control level (Feeney et al., note added in proof). Areas of hyperemia were detected in regions showing SNI, the striatum (and adjacent cortex), hippocampus, 163% and 138% of control, respectively. However, as has been noted (100), caution is required in labeling areas hyperemic or ischemic after TBI unless the metabolic demand is also measured. Amphetamine produced the expected increase in CBF in the contralateral intact hemisphere but did not alter rCBF in the areas of ischemia or hyperemia after TBI. This would indicate that amphetamine only increased CBF in areas having "normal" circulation. If increased CBF is involved in the treatment enhanced recovery discussed in this chapter, it does not act to improve circulation to the area of severe ischemia, nor does it alter areas of posttraumatic increased CBF. The enduring reduction of rCBF in the periinfarct area (39), described above, is transiently alleviated by a low dose of amphetamine (Raynaud, personal communication). Therefore, some contribution to symptom alleviation by amphetamine increases in CBF in tissue having a less severe compromised circulation may have some role in functional recovery.

Symptom Relevant Experience: NE "Enables" Physical Therapy

An important factor modifying the effect of amphetamine on functional recovery is the experience the animal receives during the period of drug evoked NE release, and this has been investigated. In the hemiplegic rat and cat, SRE (beam walk test trials) must be provided during the period of drug action for any facilitation of locomotor recovery after a single drug administration (40,41,103). Of particular interest is methylphenidate, which we initially reported had only a transient effect on functional recovery (101). Methylphenidate is the prototypical drug of the class of stimulants that block catecholamine reuptake, unlike amphetamine, which primarily produces transmitter release (102). A single dose did not produce any enduring facilitation of recovery using our standard hemiplegic rat paradigm at any dose tested. However, enduring recovery was significantly obtained using multiple doses or after a single dose by increasing SRE during the first three hours after drug administration (74). Methylphenidate may require more early beam walk test experience because of its shorter half-life compared to amphetamine. This result is of particular importance since it indicates the importance of the animal's or patient's experience during the period of NE release.

In studies of the motor system, one cannot truly control the animal's experience. One can only allow or prod the animal into making the desired movements. In experiments on vision, the experimenter has complete control over SRE. Simply turning off all lights prevents any visual experience. This has been employed to study the generality of the amphetamine + SRE treatment for promoting functional recovery after cortical injury. We measured binocular depth perception using visual cliff performance, which is lost after bilateral ablation of cortical areas 17 and 18 in the cat (104,105). This complete and "permanent" deficit can be enduringly restored after four doses of amphetamine but only if the animals are kept in the light and tested during the period of drug action, i.e., given SRE during the period of drug action. Even after seven doses of amphetamine, there is no recovery if the animals are housed in darkness for eight hours after each drug administration (104). Histochemical studies of the mitochondrial enzyme cytochrome oxidase suggest that the drug effect on binocular vision in the cat is mediated by alleviating metabolic depression in the superior colliculi (105). These data suggest that for optimal treatment of symptoms, physical therapy must be scheduled after administration of drugs increasing NE release to enhance recovery. Additionally, these studies clearly indicate that this intervention improves the ultimate level of recovery. The one clinical study omitting the critical scheduling of physical therapy to immediately after drug administration is the only report of no significant improvement of hemiplegia in stroke patients (106). Some of the other difficulties with that study have been discussed in detail following my conversations with the authors [see discussion of (106) in (60)]. Severely hemiplegic stroke patients given short-term amphetamine treatment followed in thirty minutes by intense physical therapy (PT) significantly improved motor recovery compared to placebo plus PT controls and this endured for at least ten months after stopping treatment (107).

The data reviewed indicate that the promise of the development of treatments to promote functional recovery is close to realization. Morphological and functional analysis of brain tissue, together with behavioral pharmacology data in the rat TBI model, provides insight into the mechanisms of functional recovery. Such information is leading to a synthesis of clinical and laboratory findings that is rapidly advancing our understanding of brain injury and, consequently, changing patient care.

Acknowledgments: I thank Drs. Kurt Krobert, Rob Sutherland, and Mike Wilcox for their review and discussions of an early draft of this manuscript and many helpful suggestions that improved this manuscript.

References

1. *The silent epidemic: rehabilitation of people with traumatic brain injury.* Rehab Brief, IX, 0732-2623, #4. Washington, DC: National Institute of Handicapped Research, 1988.
2. MacKenzie EJ, Shapiro S, Siegel JH. The economic impact of traumatic injuries. *JAMA* 1988;260:3290–96.
3. Lindberg R. Trauma of meninges and brain. In: Minkler J (ed.). *Pathology of the nervous system,* Vol. 2. New York: Blakston, 1968:1705–64.
4. Feeney DM, Boyeson MG, Linn RT, Murray HM, Dail WG. Responses to cortical injury: I. Methodology and local effects of contusions in the rat. *Brain Res* 1981;211:67–77.
5. Meaney DF, Ross DT, Winkelstein BA, Brasko J, Goldstein D, Bilston LB, Thibault LE, Gennarelli TA. Modification of the cortical impact model to produce axonal injury in the rat cerebral cortex. *J Neurotrauma* 1994;11: 599–612.
6. Nakano S, et al. Ischemia-induced slowly progressive neuronal damage in the rat brain. *Neuroscience* 1990;38,115–24.
7. Goldstein LB. Pharmacological interventions for improving functional tasks and altering brain behavior. This volume.
8. Sutton RL, Feeney DM. Noradrenergic pharmacotherapy and functional recovery after cortical injury. In: Illis LS (ed.). *Neurological rehabilitation.* Oxford: Blackwell Publishing Co., 1994:469–80.
9. Feeney DM, Bramlett HM, Kline AE. Neurons survive for days in contused cortex. *Neurosci Abstr* 1993;19:1881.
10. Nilsson P, Hillered L, Ponten U, Ungerstedt U. Changes in cortical extracellular levels of energy-related metabolites and amino acids following concussive brain injury. *J Cereb Blood Flow Metab* 1990;10:631–37.
11. Boyeson MG, Feeney DM, Dail WG. Cortical microstimulation thresholds adjacent to sensorimotor cortex injury. *J Neurotrauma* 1991;8:205–17.
12. Weisend MP, Feeney DM. The relationship between traumatic brain injury-induced changes in brain temperature and behavioral and anatomical outcome. *J Neurosurg* 1994;80:120–32.
13. Feeney DM, Westerberg VS. Norepinephrine and brain damage: α-noradrenergic pharmacology alters functional recovery after cortical trauma. *Can J Psychol* 1990;44:233–52.
14. Feeney DM, Sutton RL, Weisend MP, Eagan KP. Effect of delayed amphetamine treatment on primary and secondary neuropathology after cortical contusion. *Neurosci Abstr* 1990;16,779.
15. Katz RT, Brander V, Sahgal V. Updates on the diagnosis and mangement of posttraumatic hydrocephalus. *Am J Phys Med & Rehab* 1989;68:91–96.

16. Weisend MP, Feeney, DM. Effects of ketamine, halothane, and pentobarbital on locomotor recovery and cell loss following sensorimotor cortex injury. *Neurosci Abstr* 1989;15:69.

17. Feeney DM, Barela P, Heard D, Weisend MP. Secondary neuronal death and gliosis: comparison of cortical trauma, ablation and protective effects of ketamine. *J Neurotrauma* 1989;6(3):209.

18. Cortez SC, McIntosh TK, Noble LJ. Experimental fluid percussion brain injury: vascular disruption and neuronal and glial alterations. *Brain Res* 1989;482:271–82.

19. Lowenstein DH, Thomas MJ, Smith DH, McIntosh TK. Selective vulnerability of dentate hilar neurons following traumatic brain injury: a potential mechanistic link between head trauma and disorders of the hippocampus. *J Neurosci* 1992;12:4846–53.

20. Sloviter RS. Epileptic brain damage in rats induced by sustained electrical stimulation of the perforant path. I. Acute electrophysiological and light microscope studies. *Brain Res Bull* 1987;10:675–97.

21. Vicedomini JP, Nadler JV. Stimulation-induced status epilepticus: rise of the hippocampal mossy fibers in the seizures and associated neuropathology. *Brain Res* 1990;512:70–74.

22. Krobert KA, Salazar RA, Sutton RL, Feeney DM. Temporal evolution of histopathology and unit activity in rat hippocampal CA3 region after focal cortical contsuion. *J Neurotrauma* 1992;9:64.

23. Nilsson P, Ronne-Engstrom R, Fink R, Ungerstedt U, Carlson H, Hillered L. Epileptic seizure activity in the acute phase following cortical impact trauma in rat. *Brain Res* 1994;637:227–32.

24. Feeney DM, Gullotta FP, Gilmore W. Hyposexuality accompanies temporal lobe epilepsy in the cat. Under Review.

25. Feeney DM, Walker AE. The prediction of posttraumatic epilepsy: a mathematical approach. *Arch Neurol* 1979:36:8–32.

26. Feeney DM, Baron J. Diaschisis. *Stroke* 1986;17:817–30.

27. Feeney DM. Pharmacological modulation of recovery after brain injury: a reconsideration of diaschisis. *J Neuro Rehab* 1991;5:113–28.

28. Choi DW. Methods for antagonizing glutmate neurotixicity. *Cerebrovasc Brain Metab Rev* 1990;2:105–47.

29. Meldrum B. Protection against ischaemic neuronal damage by drugs acting on excitatory neurotransmission. *Cerebrovasc Brain Metab Rev* 1990;2:27–57.

30. Globus MY, et al. Ischemia induces release of glutamate in regions spared from histopathological damage in the rat. *Stroke* 1990;21(Suppl 11):1143–46.

31. Globus MY-T, Ginsberg MD, Busto R. Excitotoxic index—a biochemical marker of selective vulnerabilit. *Neurosci Lett* 1991;27:39-42.

32. Chen MJ, Rolland TM, Queen SA, Feeney DM. Modification of cerebral hypometabolism after cortical contusion: comparison of glucose utilization rates and cytochrome oxidase histochemistry. *Neurosci Abstr* 1988;14:996.

33. Hovda DA, Sutton RL, Feeney DM. Recovery of tactile placing after visual cortex ablation in cat: a behavioral and metabolic study of diaschisis. *Exp Neurol* 1987;97:1–12.

34. Yamauchi H, Fukuyama H, Kimura J. Hemodynamic and metabolic changes in crossed cerebellar hypoperfusion. *Stroke* 1992;23:855–60.

35. Transhemispheric diaschisis: a review and comment *Stroke* 1991;22:943–49.

36. Di Piero V, Chollet F, Dolan RJ, Thomas DJ, Frackowiak R. The functional nature of cerebellar diaschisis. *Stroke* 1990;21:1365-69.

37. Dail WG, Feeney DM, Murray HM, Linn RT, Boyeson G. Responses to cortical injury: II. Widespread depression of the activity of an enzyme in cortex remote from a focal injury. *Brain Res* 1981;211:79–89.

38. Lee SM, Hovda DA, Becker DP. Core of degenerating neurons in the ipsilateral parietal cortex induces spreading depression following a lateral fluid percussion injury. *Neurosci Abstr* 1994;20:846.

39. Raynaud C, Ranceutel G, Samson Y, et al. Pathophysiological study of chronic brain infarcts with I-123, Isopropl-iodo-amphetamine (IMP), the importance of the periinfarct area. *Stroke* 1987;18:21.29.

40. Feeney DM, Gonzalez A, Law WA. Amphetamine, haloperidol and experience interact to affect rate of recovery after motor cortex injury. *Science* 1982;217:855–57.

41. Hovda DA, Feeney DM. Amphetamine and experience promote recovery of function after motor cortex injury in the cat. *Brain Res* 1984;298:358–61.

42. Feeney DM, Gonzalez A, Law W. Amphetamine restores locomotor function after motor cortex injury in the rat. *Proc West Pharmacol Soc* 1981;24:15–37.

43. Feeney DM, Hovda DA. Amphetamine and apomorphine restore tactile placing after motor cortex injury in the cat. *Psychopharmacology* 1983;79: 67–71.

44. Sutton RL, Hovda DA, Feeney DM. Amphetamine accelerates functional recovery following bilateral frontal cortex ablation in cat. *Behav Neurosci* 1989;103:837–41.

45. Sanchez RJ, Krobert KA, Feeney DM. Insulin administration spares behavioral recovery after traumatic brain injury in rats. *J Neurotrauma* 1994;1:125.

46. Feeney DM, Sutton RL. Pharmacotherapy for recovery of function after brain injury. *CRC Critical Reviews in Neurobiology* 1987;3:135–97.

47. Feeney DM, Murray HM, Boyeson MG, Linn RT, Dail WG. Focal laceration and contusion of rat cerebral cortex. *Neurosci Abstr* 1979;5:510.

48. Cofer CN, Appley MH. *Motivation*. New York: John Wiley and Sons, Inc., 1968.

49. Hamm RJ, Pike BR, O'Dell DM, Lyeth BG, Jenkins LW. The rotorod test: an evaluation of its effectiveness in assessing motor deficits following traumatic brain injury. *J Neurotrauma* 1994;11:187–96.

50. Krobert KA, Feeney KA, Weiss GK. Rubrobulbar projections modify pyramidal and extrapyramidal functions during rat locomotion. *Neurosci Abstr* 1994;20:793.

51. Sutton RL, Lescaudron L, Stein DG. Behavioral consequences of moderate and severe cortical contusion in rat. *Neurosci Abstr* 1990;16:777.

52. Squire L. *Memory and brain*. New York: Oxford University Press, 1987.

53. Morris RGM, Garrud P, Rawlins J, O'Keefe J. Place navigation impaired in rats with hippocampal lesions. *Nature* 1982;319:774.

54. Smith D, Okiyama K, Thomas M, Claussen B, McIntosh TK. Evaluation of memory dysfunction following experimental brain injury using the Morris water maze. *J Neurotrauma* 1991;8:259–69.

55. Feeney DM, Weisend MP, Sutherland RJ. Traumatic brain injury causes permanent, selective learning impairments in rats. *Neurosci Abstr* 1994;20:197.

56. Sutherland RJ, Sutton RL, Feeney DM. Traumatic brain injury in the rat produces anterograde but not retrograde amnesia and impairment of hippocampal LTP. *J Neurotrauma* 1993;10:S162.

57. Sutherland R, Whishaw IQ, Kolb B. A behavioural analysis of spatial localization following electrolytic, kainate- or colchicine-induced damage to the hippocampal formation in the rat. *Behav Brain Res* 1983;7:133-53.

58. Feeney DM, Sutton RL. Catecholamines and recovery of function after brain damage. In: Sabel B, Stein D (eds.). *Pharmacological approaches to the treatment of brain and spinal cord injury*. New York: Plenum Publishing Co., 1988;121–42.

59. McIntosh T. Novel pharmacologic therapies in the treatment of experimental traumatic brain injury: a review. *J Neurotrauma* 1993;10(3):215–61.

60. Feeney DM, Weisend MP, Kline AE. Noradrenergic pharmacotherapy, intracerebral infusion and adrenal transplantation promote functional recovery after cortical damage. *J Neurotransplantation and Plasticity* 1994;4:199–214.

61. Buchan AM. Do NMDA antagonists protect against cerebral ischmia: are clinical trails warranted? *Cerebrovasc Brain Metab Rev* 1990;2:1–26.

62. Schallert T, Linder MD. Rescuing neurons from trans-synaptic degeneration after brain damage: helpful, harmful, or neural in recovery of function. *Can J Psychol* 1990;44:276–92.

63. Dietrich WD, Alonso O, Busto R, Globus MY-T, Ginsberg MD. Post-traumatic brain hypothermia reduces histopathological damage following concussive brain injury in the rat. *Acta Neuropathol* 1994;87:250–58.

64. Auer RM, Siesjö BK. Biological differences between ischemia, hypoglycemia, and epilepsy. *Ann Neurol* 1988; 24:699.707.

65. Pulsinelli WA, Waldman S, Rawlinson D, Plum F. Moderate hyperglycemia augments ischemic brain damage: a neuropathologic study in the rat. *Neurology* 1982;32:1239–46

66. Tombaugh GC, Sapolsky RM. Mechanistic distinctions between excitotoxic and acidotic hippocampal damage in an in vitro model of ischemia. *J Cereb Blood Flow Metab* 1990;-10:527–35.

67. Novelli A, Reilly JA, Lysko PG, Henneberry RC. Glutmate become neurotoxic when intracellular levels are reduced. *Brain Res* 1988;451:205–12.

68. Henneberry RC, Novelli A, Cox JA, Lysko PG. Neurotoxicity at the N-methyl-D-aspartate receptor in energy-compromised neurons. *Ann NY Acad Sci* 1989;568: 225–33.

69. Yoshino A, Hovda DA, Kawamata T, Katayama Y, Becker DP. Dynamic changes in local cerebral glucose utilization following cerebral concussion in rats: evidence of a hyper- and subsequent hypometabolic state. *Brain Res* 1991;561:106–109.

70. Hartley Z, Dubinsky JM. Changes in intracellular pH associated with glutamte excito-toxicity. *J Neurosci* 1993;13:4690–99.

71. Marie C, Bralet J. (1991) Blood glucose level and morphological brain damage following cerebral ischemia. *Cerebrovasc Brain Metab Rev* 1991;3:29–38.

72. Salo AA, Feeney DM. Reduction of morbidity, mortality, and lesion size in rat model of cerebral infarction with amphetamine. *Soc Neurosci Abst* 1987;13:1268.

73. Chen MJ, Sutton RL, Feeney DM. Recovery of function following brain injury in rat and cat: beneficial effects of phenylpropanolamine. *Neurosci Abstr* 1986;12:881.

74. Nishino K, Kowoda M, Ito TL.-DOPS facilitated motor recovery in rat model and chronic stroke cases, *Neurosci Abstr.*

75. Boyeson MG, Harmon RL. Effects of trazodone and desipramine on motor recovery in brain injured rats. *Am J Phys Med Rehab* 1993;72:286–93.

76. Sutton RL, Feeney DM. α-noradrenergic agonists and antagonists affect recovery and maintenance of beam-walking ability after sensorimotor cortex ablation in the rat. *Rest Neurol Neurosci* 1992;4: 1–11.

77. Hovda DA, Feeney DM, Salo AA. Phenoxybenzamine but not haloperidol reinstates all motor and sensory deficits in cats fully recovered from sensorimotor cortex ablations. *Neuro Abstr* 1983;9:1002.

78. Feeney DM, Hovda DA, Salo AA. Phenoxybenzamine reinstates all motor and sensory deficits in cats fully recovered from sensorimotor cortex ablations. *Federation Proceedings* 1983;42:1157.

79. Feeney DM, Boyeson MG, Hovda DA, Salo AA. Catecholamines affect recovery from brain injury. 5th CA Symposium, Goteburg, Sweden, 1983, 146, 133–34. *Abstract in Progress in Neuro-Psychopharmacology and Biological Psychiatry* (Suppl), p.133, 1983.

80. Sutton RL, Feeney DM. Yohimbine accelerates recovery and clonidine and prazosin reinstate deficits after recovery in rats with sensorimotor cortex ablation. *Neurosci Abstr* 1987;13:913.

81. Goldstein LB, Davis JN. Clonidine impairs recovery of beam-walking after a sensorimotor cortex lesion in the rat. *Brain Res* 1990;508:305–309.

82. Goldstein LB, Poe HV, Davis JN. An animal model of recovery of function after stroke: facilitation of recovery an α2-adrenergic antagonist. *Ann Neurol* 1989; 26:157–59.

83. Boyeson MG, Feeney DM. Intraventricular norepinephrine facilitates recovery following sensorimotor cortex injury. *Pharmacology, Biochemistry and Behavior* 1990;35: 497–501.

84. Sutton RL, Hovda DA, Feeney DM. Intracerebral chomaffin cell autografts accelerate locomotor recovery and reinstate tactile placing in adult cats with unilateral frontal cortex ablation. *Brain Dysfunction* 1989; 2:201–10.

85. Boyeson MG, Feeney DM. Adverse effects of catecholaminergic agonists and antagonists on recovery of locomotor ability following unilateral cerebellar ablations. *Rest Neurol Neurosci* 1991;3:227–33.

86. Boyeson MG, Krobert KA. Cerebellar norepinephrine infusions facilitate recovery after sensorimotor cortex injury. *Brain Res Bull* 1992;29:435–39.

87. Boyeson MG, Krobert KA, Scherer PJ, Grade, CM. Reinstatement of motor deficits in recovered brain injured animals. *Rest Neurol Neurosci* 1993;5:283–90.

88. Feeney DM, Sutton RL, Boyeson MG, Hovda DA, Dail WG. The locus coeruleus and cerebral metabolism: recovery of function after cortical injury. *Physiological Psychology* 1985:13:197–203.

89. Krobert K, Feeney DM. Effects of amphetamine on biogenic amine levels following right sensorimotor cortex ablation in rat. *Neurosci Abstr* 1990; 16:43.

90. Prasad MR, Ramaih C, McIntosh TK, Dempsey RJ, Hipkins S, Yurek D. Regional levels of lactate and norepinephrine after experimental brain injury. *J Neurochem* 1994;63:1086–94.

91. Krobert KA, Sutton RL, Feeney DM. Spontaneous and amphetamine evoked release of noradrenalin after cortical contusion. *J Neurochem* 1994;62:2233–40.

92. Goldstein LB. Acute unilateral sensorimotor injury in the rat blocks d-amphetamine induced norepinephrine release in cerebellum. *Rest Neurol Neurosci* 1993;5:371–77.

93. Prasad MR, Tzigaret CM, Smith D, Soares H, McIntosh TK. Decreased α1 adrenergic receptors after experimental brain injury. *J Neurotrauma* 1992; 9:269–79.

94. Levin BE, Pan S, Dunn Maynell A. Chronic alterations in rat adrenoceptors following traumatic brain injury. *Rest Neurol Neurosci* 1994;7:5–12.

95. Hurwitz BE, Dietrich WD, McCabe PM, Alonso O, Watson BD, Ginsberg MD, Schneiderman N. Amphetamine promotes recovery from sensory-motor integration deficit after thrombotic infarction of the primary somatosensory rat cortex. *Stroke* 1991;22(5): 648–54.

96. Dietrich WD, Alonso O, Busto R, Ginsberg MD. The effect of amphetamine on functional brain activation in normal and post-infarcted rat. *Stroke* 1990;21(Suppl 3):147–50.

97. Kogure K, Scheinberg P, Kishikawa H, Utsunomiya Y, Busto R. Adrenergic control of cerebral blood flow and energy metabolism in the rat. *Stroke* 1979;10:179–84.

98. Minneman KP, Johnson D. Characterization of α₁ adrenergic receptors linked to inositol metabolism in rat cerebral cortex. *J Pharm Exp Therapeutics* 1984;230:317–22.

99. Subbarao, K.V. and Hertz, L. Stimulation of energy metabolism by α1 adrenergic agonists in primary cultures of astrocytes. *J Neurosci Res* 1991;28:399–405.

100. Le HM, Lifshitz J, Smith ML, Pinanong P, Lee SM, Becker DP, Hovda DA. Uncoupling of glucose metabolism and blood flow in degenerating cortical and hippocampal areas following unilateral cortical contusion. *Neurosci Abstr* 1994;20:196.

101. Kline AE, Chen MJ, Tso-Oliveras DY, Feeney DM. Methylphenidate treatment following ablation induced hemiplegia: experience during drug action alters effects on recovery of function. *Pharmacology Biochemistry and Behavior* 1994;48:773–79.

102. Scheel-Kruger J. Comparative studies of various amphetamine analogues demonstrating different interactions with the metabolism of the catecholamines in the brain. *European J Pharmacol* 1971;14: 47–59.

103. Goldstein LB, Davis JN. Post-lesion practice and amphetamine-facilitated recovery of beam-walking in the rat. *Beh Neurosci* 1990;104: 318–25.

104. Feeney DM, Hovda DA. Reinstatement of binocular depth perception by amphetamine and visual experience after visual cortex ablation. *Brain Res* 1985;342:352–56.

105. Hovda DA, Sutton RL, Feeney DM. Amphetamine-induced recovery of visual cliff performance after bilateral visual cortex ablation in cats: measurements of depth perception thresholds. *Beh Neuosci* 1989;103,:574–84.

106. Borucki SJ, Landberg J, Reding M. The effect of dextromethorphan on motor recovery after stroke. *Neurology* 1992;42(Suppl 3):329.

107. Walker-Batson D, Smith P, Curtis S, Unwin H, Greenlee R. Amphetamine paired with physical therapy accelerates motor recovery after stroke. *Stroke* 1995;26:2254-59.

NOTES ADDED IN PROOF

1. Feeney DM, Weisend MP. Neuronal death in thalamic nuclei Lateralis Dorsalis and Reticularis ipsilateral to traumatic sensorimotor cortex injury. *Neuroscience Abstracts* 1995, 21.

2. The first Internet virtual meeting in Neuroscience. The title is Symposium on Brain Damage and Functional Recovery Poster EE0505, "Mechanisms of Delayed Cell Death in Cortical Contusions" Feeney DM, Scremin OU, Ni S, Kline AE, Wilcox MJ on the World Wide Web at http://spine.unm.edu/neurosurg/sym/welcome3.html mirrored in Japan at: http://www.medic.mie-u.ac.jp/2NDCNG/BRAIND/WELCOME3.HTML.

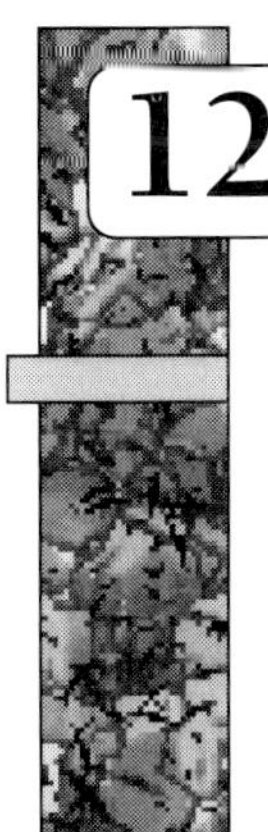

12

The Effect of Strategy on Cognitive Processing: Evidence from Pure Alexia

H. Branch Coslett, M.D.

The mechanisms underlying recovery of function after central nervous system insults remain obscure. One often invoked but rarely documented mechanism by which recovery may occur is that subjects adapt to cerebral dysfunction—either consciously or unconsciously—by employing different cognitive strategies. In this chapter, I present data which I believe demonstrate that the use of different information processing strategies may alter the performance of patients with brain lesions. Additionally, I suggest that, at least in some instances, alternate strategies may be mediated by different brain structures.

The data regarding the effect of strategies on performance come from five patients with the syndrome of "pure alexia" or "alexia without agraphia." This disorder, first described by Déjérine in 1892 (1), is characterized by the inability to read aloud or for comprehension in the absence of aphasia, agraphia, or dementia. As this disorder is typically observed on association with a left occipital lobe infarction that causes a right homonymous hemianopia as well as a disruption of the forceps major carrying visual information from the preserved right hemisphere to the left hemisphere language processing centers, pure alexia has traditionally been attributed to a "disconnection" of visual information in the right hemisphere from the left hemisphere peri-Sylvian structures, which subserve language.

When instructed to read a word, subjects with pure alexia often resort to a serial letter naming strategy; using this letter-by-letter approach, for example, a pure alexic may identify the word "dog" by first naming the constituent letters aloud and then naming the word on the basis of the letter names. Recently, however, my colleague Eleanor Saffran and I [(2,3); see also Landis et al., 1980] have demonstrated that at least some patients with pure alexia are able to derive information from words without using a letter-by-letter strategy; in fact these patients appear to read implicitly as they may be unable to explicitly identify the words and, indeed, often claim not to have seen the word. In the following section we first present data demonstrating that these subjects do indeed exhibit implicit reading. Subsequently, we present data suggesting that letter-by-letter reading and implicit reading reflect the operation of two distinct reading strategies.

Subjects

We report data from five subjects with pure alexia; details of the history, examination, and lesion localization for four of the subjects (JG, TL, JC, AF) may be found in Coslett et al. (2). Clinical information for the fifth subject (JWC) may be found in Coslett and Saffran (3). Briefly, all subjects were right-handed and developed pure alexia after suffering ischemic infarctions involving the left occipital lobe or, in the case of JG, the left lateral geniculate and the splenium of the corpus callosum. All subjects exhibited letter-by-letter reading; as a consequence of this laborious, serial letter naming strategy, all five subjects demonstrated an effect of word length, tending to be slower and less accurate when reading longer words (see Table 12-1).

Lexical Decision Tests

Although Déjérine (1) and subsequently Geschwind (5) had suggested that the right (non-dominant) hemisphere is "word-blind," a number of lines of evidence including evaluations of "deep dyslexics" and patients after corpus callostomy have suggested that the right hemisphere maintains the capacity to read at least some types of words; if the right hemisphere is indeed literate, one might ask why pure alexics do not utilize the capacity of the right hemisphere to read. One possible explanation for the failure of pure dyslexics to read is that reading is typically assumed to entail the explicit, overt naming of the stimulus. Because reading is assumed to necessarily entail overt word naming, we suggest, subjects employ a serial letter naming strategy which, even if inefficient and error prone, produces explicit responses.

In light of this consideration, we reasoned that if we were to demonstrate the reading capacity of the right hemisphere, we would have to test patients under conditions that prevented them from employing the preferred letter-by-letter strategy. To accomplish this objective, we used a microcomputer to present stimuli for a brief interval, thereby preventing patients from relying on the slow letter-by-letter strategy.

The first experiment to be described here was a lexical decision test in which patients are shown a letter string containing three, four, or five letters and asked to indicate if the letter comprised a real word (e.g., "roof") or a non-word (e.g., "slet").

Table 12-1. *Speed of Oral Reading As a Function of Word Length (in Seconds)*

Patient	Number of Letters				
	3	4	5	6	7
JG	9	13	17	27	28
TL	2	3	3	5	4
JC	2	6	17	16	30
AF	31	83	—	—	—
JWC	16	21	26	26	60

Stimuli included sixty high frequency words (mean frequency of 445.8 counts/million), sixty low frequency words (all 2 count/million), sixty word-like non-words (e.g., "shart"), and sixty non-words with unusual or illegal orthographic sequences (e.g., "twilk"). Patients were told that the letter string would be presented briefly and were instructed not to try to name the word but to say "yes" if the letter string was a real word.

Despite instructions to refrain from naming the words, patients frequently tried in vain to respond on the basis of partial letter information (e.g., the fact that the first letter was an "s"). When letter names were reported, patients were repeatedly admonished to avoid a letter-by-letter strategy but to attempt to "see the whole word" or get a "feeling" or "impression"about the letter string.

The results, expressed as the percentage of "yes" responses, are presented in Table 12-2. All patients were more accurate with high frequency words compared to low frequency words and with improbable words compared to word-like non-words. Furthermore, although far from perfect, analysis with a "d" statistic revealed that all subjects distinguished words from non-words with an accuracy that exceeded chance. Note that this effect was not attributable to a partial preservation of the ability to read explicitly. Patients rarely explicitly identified words and, in fact, claimed not to have seen the letter string more frequently than they correctly identified the word. Deleting the trials on which the patients explicitly identified the word did not alter the effect for any patient.

Word Comprehension

Having demonstrated that all five patients were able to reliably, if imperfectly, distinguish words from non words in the absence of explicit identification, a series of experiments was performed to assess the ability of the patients to derive semantic information from words that they were unable to name.

In the first study, a single word was again briefly presented with a microcomputer. In this task, however, patients were asked to indicate whether the word was

Table 12-2. *Lexical Decision at Brief Exposures*

| | | % "Yes" Responses | | | | | | |
| | | Words | | | Non-words | | | |
Patient	Exp. ms	Hi Freq N = 60	Lo Freq N = 60	Hi + Lo N = 120	Hi – N N = 120	Lo – N N = 60	Hi + Lo N = 120	d′
JG	250	75	37	56	35	25	30	0.68*
TL	150	82	78	80	63	38	50	0.84*
JC	250	78	52	65	28	11	19	1.30*
AΓ	250	80	53	67	42	18	30	0.96*
JWC	242	93	48	71	57	43	45	0.55*

p <.05.

an animal name. Stimuli for the experiment included twenty-five animal names (e.g., "mouse"), twenty-five words judged to be visually similar to the animal names (e.g., "mount"), and twenty-five words that were not visually similar to the animal names (e.g., "rally"). The three groups of stimuli were matched for length and frequency. The three types of stimuli were presented in random sequence.

In a second study, the target words were names of food items; as in the previous experiment, there were twenty-five names of edible items (e.g., "chocolate"), twenty-five visually similar words (e.g., "chockfull"), and twenty-five words matched for length and frequency but with no visual or semantic similarity to the target words.

For both studies, patients were instructed to attend to the whole word and derive a "feeling" or impression about the word. Letter-by-letter reading was discouraged by the examiners. Patients were told that it was not important to identify words but that they should report those words that they thought they had identified.

The data for the five patients on both tasks are presented in Table 12-3. Once again, patients were far from perfect in their responses but all subjects performed significantly better than chance ($p < .05$). Two patients failed to explicitly identify even a single word, whereas three patients correctly named between 1.3% and 6.7% of words. Interestingly, although unable to name the word, patients occasionally indicated that they had a feel for the word and offered a brief comment; examples of these responses included *lobster*—"lives in water," *oyster*—"funny name, body flat, like a duckbill, lives in water," and *rabbit*—"has big ears, something about Easter."

Additional tests requiring patients to match words presented for a brief interval with a microcomputer to one of two line drawings presented free-field provided similar results: although not perfect, all five patients performed well above chance.

Thus, converging data from these experiments demonstrate that all five subjects were able to derive the meaning of words that they were unable to explicitly identify.

Evidence for Different Reading Strategies

One possible explanation for the pattern of performance demonstrated by these five patients is that they were able to derive information about the form and meaning of a letter string by means of at least two different procedures. The first involves serial let-

Table 12-3. *Category Decision at Brief Exposures*

		% Correct	
		Animal?	Edible?
Patient	Exp. ms	N = 75	N = 75
JG	250	75	80
TL	100	69	67
JC	250	85	79
AF	250	71	76
JWC	249	73	76

ter naming on the basis of which the patient is able to explicitly identify the word. The second may involve access to stored word forms and semantics in the absence of explicit word identification, a process that, as we have suggested, may be mediated by the right hemisphere. To test the hypothesis that two distinct and possible incompatible procedures are available to these patients, we performed an additional study in one of our recent patients, JWC (3).

We reasoned that if JWC utilized one procedure for purposes of word naming but a different procedure to access meaning for briefly displayed words, his performance with the same stimuli would differ as a function of task demands. That is, in the context of the studies described previously, we predicted that when asked to explicitly identify words he would be able to name a proportion of the stimuli using slow, laborious letter-by-letter strategy but would perform poorly on semantic judgment tasks for those stimuli he was unable to name. In contrast, when asked to make a semantic judgment, JWC would be expected to perform well above chance but would be unable to explicitly name the words that he had correctly classified. These predictions were tested in a session in which stimulus duration and patient instructions were varied.

The first task in this session was to indicate whether a rapidly presented word was a male or female name. Thirty names (sixteen male, fourteen female) were presented in random sequence for 249 ms. using the microcomputer. Although he was unable to explicitly identify any names, JWC responded correctly on all thirty trials. The second task was the animal categorization test described previously, which had last been administered to the patient seven weeks prior. JWC was told that the primary task was to determine if the briefly presented word was the name of an animal; he was also instructed to name any words that he believed he had identified. He responded correctly on 85% of trials (64/75) while naming only four words.

In the next task, an attempt was made to induce JWC to switch from a reading strategy affording access to semantics to a strategy providing explicit word identity. To this end, he was asked to explicitly name sets of five words containing three-, four-, five-, and six-letter words printed on 5 × 7 inch cards. Stimuli were presented for an unlimited period and the interval from word presentation to response was recorded. JWC was pathologically slow in word identification, requiring nineteen seconds on average to correctly read a five-letter word. Additionally, a clear effect of length was noted, suggesting that JWC employed a serial letter naming strategy.

Next, a second task requiring strict word identification was performed. Stimuli for this task include the seventy-five words from the "edible" semantic categorization task described previously. On this administration, however, JWC was told that each letter string would be presented for 2,000 ms. and that his primary objective was to *name* the word. He was also told that if unable to name the word, he would be asked if the word designated something that could be eaten. It was clearly emphasized to JWC that word identification was the primary task. As seen in Table 12-3, JWC correctly named sixteen of twenty-five food items but was unable to explicitly name any of the visually similar or unrelated words; overall, then, JWC correctly named 21% of words presented for two seconds. Most errors involved the reporting of a food name.

Performance on the judgment task was also analyzed. JWC responded correctly on only thirty-nine of seventy-five trials (52%). Additionally, excluding those trials on which he offered an explicit response, he responded correctly on only twenty-two of forty-three trials (51%). Thus, when asked to explicitly identify words, JWC performed at chance in judging whether or not the referent of the target word is edible.

Finally, to ensure that JWC's poor performance with semantic judgments was not attributable to specific visual or semantic features of the stimuli, a randomized version of the same stimuli was presented once again after a rest period. On this occasion, however, the patient was told that the stimuli would be presented for a very brief interval and that his major objective was to determine if the referent of the word was edible. He was told to name the word if he could but that explicit identification was not the major goal. JWC correctly indicated if the stimulus designated an edible item on sixty-five of seventy-five trials (87%), a performance that is far better than chance. He correctly identified only four of the seventy-five stimuli.

Overall, the patient's performance on these tasks conforms to the predictions outlined previously. When asked to explicitly identify words, JWC accurately reported 21% of words presented for two seconds; he reported one or more letters on all trials, suggesting that he was employing a letter-by-letter strategy. When using this letter naming strategy, he performed at chance at semantic categorization. In contrast, when instructed to make a semantic judgment about briefly presented words, he performed well on three tasks, including one on which he had performed at chance when emphasis was placed on word identification. While focusing on semantic categorization, he explicitly identified only 5% of words and never reported partial letter information.

Summary and Conclusions

We have presented data from five patients who lost the ability to read fluently after infarctions in the posterior portions of the left hemisphere. All five patients initially attempted to read by means of a slow, effortful, and efficient letter-by-letter strategy

Table 12-4. *Performance As a Function of Task Type (JWC)*

Task Order	Task	Exposure	N	% Correct
1	Categorization male or female name?	249 ms	30	100
2	Categorization animal?	249 ms	75	85
3	Name word	Unlimited		100
4	Name, then edible?	2,000 ms	25 foods 25 vis. foils 25 unrel. foils	51
5	Categorization edible?	249 ms	25 foods 25 vis. foils 25 unrel. foils	86

that afforded explicit identification of some words; using this strategy, word meaning was accessed only after word naming. We subsequently demonstrated that when forced to abandon the letter-by-letter strategy by brief stimulus exposure, all five patients demonstrated access to information about the meaning and lexical status of letter strings (that is, whether it is a word or not) that they were unable to explicitly report.

The hypothesis that the patients employed different reading strategies—a letter-by-letter strategy with unlimited exposure and a "whole-word" strategy with brief stimulus presentation—was directly supported in testing with one patient. JWC identified 21% of words displayed for two seconds when asked to name the word but performed at chance on semantic judgment tasks for those words he was unable to explicitly identify. In contrast, when instructed to perform a semantic judgment task, he performed significantly better than chance but named only 5% of stimuli.

The data presented here demonstrate that differences in information processing strategies may indeed significantly influence the performance of patients with brain lesions. More generally, these data suggest that comprehensive accounts of recovery of function must consider not only phenomena such as neuronal plasticity and pharmacological effects on brain function but also the mechanisms by which patient strategies modulate brain function.

Acknowledgments: This research was supported in part by NIH grants NS26400 and NS00876. The author would like to acknowledge the major contributions of Eleanor M. Saffran, Ph.D., to the research reported here.

References

1. Déjérine J. *Contribution a l'etude anatomo-pathologique et clinique des differentes varietes de cecite verbale. Comptes Rendus Hebdomadaires des Seances et Memoires de la Societe de Biologie,* Ninth series 1892;4:61–90.
2. Coslett HB, Saffran EM. Evidence for preserved reading in pure alexia. *Brain* 1989;112.327–29.
3. Coslett HB, Saffran EM, Greenbaum S, Schwartz H. Reading in pure alexia. the effect of strategy. *Brain* 1993;116:21–37.
4. Landis T, Regard M, Serrat A. Iconic reading in a case of alexia without agraphia caused by a brain tumor: a tachistoscopic study. *Brain and Language* 1980;11:45–53.
5. Geschwind N. Disconnection syndromes in animals and man. *Brain* 1965;88:237–94, 585–644.

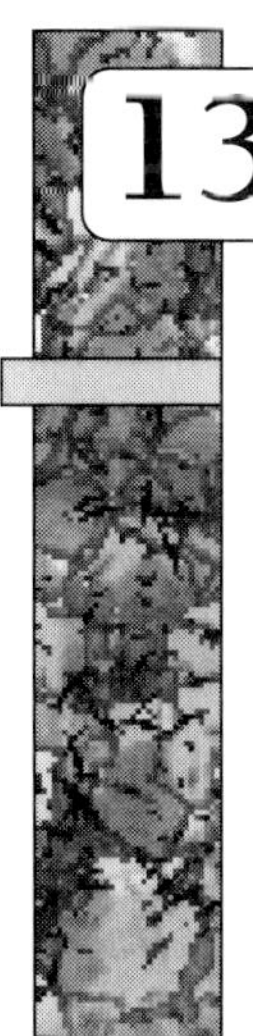

Effects of Motor Restriction of an Unimpaired Upper Extremity and Training on Improving Functional Tasks and Altering Brain Behaviors

Edward Taub, Ph.D., Rama D. Pidikiti, M.D.
Stephanie C. DeLuca, B.A., and Jean E. Crago, M.S., P.T.

This chapter outlines a new approach to the rehabilitation of upper extremity movement in chronic stroke patients. In particular, it describes a set of specific protocols that can be used to produce a substantial increase in the amount that an affected extremity is used in the life situation by patients selected by the inclusion criteria used in our project. The patients we have worked with had experienced a stroke from one year to many years prior to admission to the project. According to the traditional view in the field, stroke patients with this degree of chronicity should have reached a plateau in their motor improvement from which they will not recover further function. In apparent contrast, many clinicians have had the experience of observing some chronic stroke patients who could be brought to exhibit substantial improvement in motor capacity with appropriate therapy and careful training. The almost invariable problem with this improvement is that it is limited to the clinic. In a figure of speech that the present authors have heard repeated by a number of clinicians, the improvement is often lost as they watch the patient walk across the clinic threshold and into the adjacent hall. The patient rapidly reverts to the degraded motor pattern that had just been laboriously and successfully improved. The present authors have searched the literature without being able to find mention of this commonly observed phenomenon, perhaps both because explicit studies have never been carried out with respect to it and because irregularly observed treatment failures do not lend themselves easily to description in a systematic publication. However, the frustration involved in repeatedly seeing one's apparent therapeutic successes turn into failures is often cited in informal conversation as a contributor to therapist "burnout."

During the course of this century, there have been a small number of investigators who have reported the use of training techniques that have resulted in some improvements in limb use in chronic stroke patients whose greatly impaired motor function was presumably not amenable to further recovery (1,2). Indeed, Paul Bach-y-Rita and his colleagues operated a ward for some years at the University of Wisconsin School of Medicine for treatment of chronic stroke and head injury patients. Their program was characterized by the consistent application of therapeutic procedures in the clinic in conjunction with a strong emphasis on the establishment of an individually tailored home practice regimen. The program is reported to have produced long-term improvement in the motor function of many of these patients, who by traditional criteria would not otherwise have changed in motor status (3–5).

These results have been noted by the physical medicine community, but they have achieved little actual penetration into clinical practice. The reason for this is probably two-fold. First, it is contrary to the personal experience of most clinicians that chronic stroke patients can achieve substantial *long-term* improvement in motor ability, even with the administration of consistent and well-executed physical therapy, except in isolated cases. Claims to the contrary, even though they are based on the administration of new therapies or significant variations of older therapies, tend to be met by skepticism. Second, the reports of therapeutic success with chronic stroke patients have not been accompanied by descriptions of clear-cut, explicit protocols that a potentially interested clinician could employ. The lack of a standardized protocol probably discourages attempts at replication based primarily on published papers.

With regard to these issues, the approach to the rehabilitation of movement to be described below has several features that have clinical relevance. One of the salient characteristics of the approach is that it focuses primary interest on translation of the motor gains made in the clinic to increased use of the affected extremity in the life situation. This is accomplished by a variety of means, but most importantly through the use of a restraint or constraint device that forces or strongly promotes the use of the affected extremity outside the clinic, without requiring the special cooperation of the patient other than compliance in wearing the device. Additionally, the protocols to be described are clear-cut and standardized. It is our experience that optimal results can be achieved by tailoring the treatment program in the clinic to each patient's specific deficits. However, very good results can be achieved using an unvarying, straightforward protocol. In particular, the procedure for accomplishing transfer of clinic improvement to the life situation (the constraint devices) is the same for all patients using the two recommended treatments.

To date, we have worked with seventeen experimental and five attention-control subjects meeting the project's inclusion criteria. All experimental subjects exhibited significant and large improvements in use of the affected upper extremity. None of the control subjects exhibited long-term motor improvement; two of them showed a modest short-term improvement, which did not persist past the first month post-treatment. Nevertheless, the number of subjects tested is relatively small to date. Although other laboratories have obtained results similar to ours using some of the techniques to be described (6–12), there is clearly a need for replication in still other laboratories and with a large number of subjects. Until this is accomplished, our results must be considered suggestive and not in any way conclusive.

Our work with chronic stroke patients (13) is based directly on studies carried out with monkeys given somatosensory deafferentation of a single extremity (14). We have simply transferred the techniques developed in this basic research to the human case after stroke. Additionally, the efficacy of our techniques is explained as being based on the operation of a mechanism termed *learned nonuse.* Our techniques are thought to work because they overcome learned nonuse (14,15). Thus, before presenting the data from human patients, it would be of value to first describe the somatosensory deafferentation research with monkeys and the concept of overcoming learned nonuse derived from this research.

Research with Monkeys

By severing all the dorsal roots innervating a limb, one eliminates all sensation from that limb involved in the support of ongoing behavior sequences, while leaving the motor innervation intact over the ventral roots. When a single forelimb is deafferented in a monkey, the animal stops making use of it in the free situation. This was the classic observation of Mott and Sherrington (16) and others (17–19). My co-workers and I found that it was possible to induce a monkey to use the deafferented limb by two general types of techniques.

One technique involved restriction of movement of the *intact* upper extremity through the use of a device that left the deafferented limb free (19,20). Use of the deafferented limb would usually begin within an hour after the restriction device had been secured, often for postural support while the animal was in a sitting position. The period of postoperative nonuse of the affected extremity could often be of years-long duration; nevertheless, within several hours the limb could typically be used, although somewhat clumsily, for a wide variety of activities, including ambulation, climbing, and even thumb-forefinger prehension of small objects. When the animals were removed from the movement restriction device shortly after exhibiting purposive use of the deafferented extremity, they immediately reverted to nonuse of that limb. However, if they were left in the device for a period of time, typically one week (although for one animal it was a period as short as three days), the use of the deafferented limb persisted after the device was removed with no apparent diminution of range or quality of movement. Moreover, use of the limb was permanent, being observed for the remainder of the animals' lives, which in one case was over four years (14,15). In this fashion, a useless limb was converted into a limb that could be used extensively.

A second method for overcoming the inability to use a single deafferented limb was found to be the application of procedures for training that limb. In initial work, conditioned response techniques were employed for enabling the animals to make one of a variety of movements with the deafferented limb in order to either avoid an electric shock or to obtain food or liquid when hungry or thirsty, respectively. The required movements included phasic forelimb flexion (19,21–23) grasp (24), sus tained forelimb flexion (14,15), and compensation for progressively increasing loads on the arm (14,15,25,26). However, transfer never occurred between the experimental and life situations (14,15). The movements that were trained in the conditioning chamber were never observed to be performed in the colony environment.

The conditioned response paradigm is, of course, just one type of training technique. An even more effective training method for inducing recovery of motor function was found to be shaping, in which a desired motor or behavioral objective is approached in small steps, by successive approximations (27–31). With shaping techniques, the animals not only learned to employ a single deafferented limb in the training situation, but its use transferred to the life situation as well. This was in contrast to the case for conditioned response training. Shaping appeared to provide a bridge from the training situation, enabling extensive movement in the animal's normal environment. The behaviors shaped included (1) pointing at visual targets (32), and (2) prehension in juveniles, deafferented on day of birth (33) and prenatally (34), who had never exhibited any prehension previously. In both cases, shaping permitted an almost complete reversal of the motor disability, which progressed from total absence of the target behavior to very good (although not normal) performance. This can be characterized as a substantial rehabilitation of movement.

■■■■■*A Possible Mechanism: Learned Nonuse and Constraint-Induced Facilitation of Movement*

The authors offer the following analysis to provide a hypothesis to explain why the techniques described in this article might be effective. In the event that the hypothesis is incorrect, this would not have been the practical effect of reducing whatever clinical efficaciousness the techniques have been shown to have. Moreover, the authors recognize that even if the proposed mechanism is correct in essence, the actual method by which it operates is unlikely to be exactly as specified. Various important modulating influences have not been taken into consideration in the preliminary formulation. These include site and laterality of lesion, extent of lesion, interaction with other mechanisms, and environmental influences. However, it is considered to be of value to offer the tentative formulation as a stimulus for empirical test and further hypothesis information.

Several converging lines of evidence suggested that nonuse of a single deafferented limb is a learning phenomenon involving a conditioned suppression of movement. [For a description of the experimental analysis leading to this conclusion, see Taub (14,15).] The restraint and training techniques appeared to be effective because they overcome the learned nonuse.

As background, one should note that substantial neurological injury usually leads to a shock-like phenomenon, whether at the level of the spinal cord (spinal shock) or brain (diaschisis or cortical shock). With regard to deafferentation, the elimination of somatosensory input results initially in a reduction within the spinal cord in the background level of excitation that maintains neurons in a subliminal state of readiness to respond. This effect is most marked in the deafferented segments of the spinal cord, where the depressed condition of motoneurons greatly elevates the threshold for incoming excitation necessary to produce movement. The early post-surgical spinal shock may also be partly due to active inhibitory processes. As time elapses following deafferentation, recovery processes, which are at present incompletely understood, raise the background level of excitability of motoneurons so that movements can once again, *at least potentially,* be expressed. The period of spinal shock in adolescent monkeys lasts from two to six months following forelimb deafferentation (14,15,35).

Thus, immediately after operation, the monkeys cannot use a deafferented limb; recovery from spinal shock requires considerable time. An animal with one deafferented limb tries to use that extremity in the early postoperative period, but it cannot. It gets along reasonably well in the laboratory environment on three limbs and is therefore rewarded for this pattern of behavior, which consequently increases in strength. Moreover, continued attempts to use the deafferented limb often lead to aversive consequences, such as incoordination and falling, and, in general, failure in any activity attempted with the deafferented limb. Many learning experiments have demonstrated that aversive consequences (punishment) result in the suppression of behavior. The habit of nonuse persists, and consequently the monkeys never learn that the limb had become potentially useful several months after operation. This combined reward of a degraded, compensatory behavior pattern and the suppression of behavior produced by punishment may be characterized as a learned nonuse. The mechanism is depicted schematically in Figure 13-1.

When the movements of the intact limb are restricted several months after unilateral deafferentation, the situation changes dramatically. The animal either uses the deafferented limb or it cannot with any degree of efficiency feed itself, locomote, or carry out a large portion of its normal activities of daily life. This new constraint on behavior increases the motivation to use the limb and induces the monkey to do so (depicted schematically in Figure 13-2).

The conditioned response and shaping situations also involve placing major constraints on the animal's behavior. In the conditioning chamber, if the monkeys do not

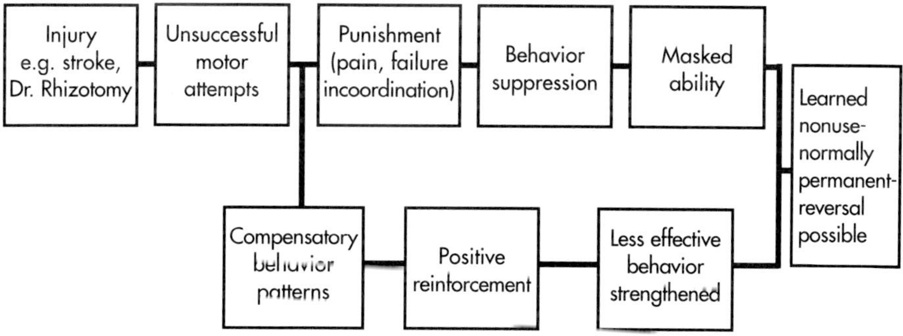

Figure 13-1. Schematic model for development of learned nonuse. After Tries (10).

perform the required response, they either receive electric shock or do not receive food pellets or liquid when hungry or thirsty, respectively. Similarly, during shaping, hunger and the need to make an improved movement place a new requirement on behavior. The animals can not "get along" in either situation using just the intact forelimb, as they can in the colony environment.

Thus, the movement restriction, conditioned response, and shaping situations share a common feature; each involves a constraint-induced facilitation of impaired improvement that has the effect of overcoming the learned nonuse. This would appear to be the mechanism responsible in each case for enabling the remediation of motor ability.

All the evidence cited until now constitutes indirect evidence for the learned nonuse hypothesis. Consequently, an attempt was made to test the hypothesis in direct fashion (14,15). This involved restricting the movements of a deafferented limb in several animals so that they could not attempt to use it for a period of three months following surgery. The reasoning was that in thus preventing an animal from trying to use the deafferented limb during the period before spinal shock had passed and recovery of neural excitability had taken place, one should thereby prevent the animal from learning that the limb could not be used during that interval. Learned nonuse of the deafferented limb should therefore not develop. Thus, after the restraint is removed three months postoperatively the animal should be able to use the deafferented extremity in the free situation, although never again subjected to restriction of the intact limb. The results were in conformity with this prediction. On removal from the restraining device, it was found that the animals were able to use the deafferented limb and the ability to do so spontaneously reached the level normally exhibited by animals given prolonged restriction of the intact limb in the work discussed previously. Suggestive evidence was also obtained during the course of deafferentation experiments carried out in early life and prenatally (14).

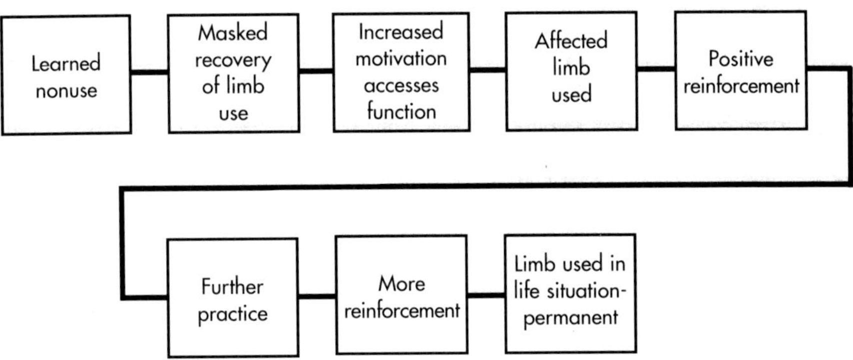

Figure 13-2. Schematic model of mechanism for overcoming learned nonuse.

Applicability of the Model to Human Patients After Stroke

During the course of this century, several investigators have found that a behavioral technique could be employed in nonhuman animals to substantially improve a motor deficit resulting from neurological damage other than deafferentation (36–39). There may thus be some interesting parallels between the possible participation of a learned nonuse mechanism in the masking of the motor capacity actually present both after pyramidotomy and other motor lesions and after unilateral deafferentation.

Given the general nature of the learned nonuse mechanism, it was reasoned that constraint-induced overcoming of learned nonuse might be an appropriate approach for the rehabilitation of motor impairments due to injury to the nervous system in humans. For example, stroke in humans often leaves patients with an apparently permanent loss of function in an upper extremity, although the limb is not paralyzed. Additionally, the motor deficit is preponderantly unilateral. These factors are similar to those that pertain to the situation after unilateral forelimb deafferentation in monkeys. Therefore, it seemed reasonable to formulate a formal protocol that simply transferred the techniques used for converting a useless limb to one that could be used extensively from unilaterally deafferented monkeys to human patients who had experienced a cerebrovascular accident (CVA) (14).

A question might arise as to whether a mechanism that leads to rehabilitation of movement after somatosensory deafferentation would have relevance to the rehabilitation of movement after stroke since the two involve very different types of damage to the nervous system. Somatosensory deafferentation involves the interruption of afferent neurons at spinal cord level, while the motor deficit after stroke results from the destruction of motor and other neurons at cortical level. However, both deafferentation and stroke are similar in that both are followed by a period of central nervous system (CNS) shock. The learned nonuse mechanism is predicated on this phenomenon.

CNS shock is usually not permanent, although recovery from it is gradual. If a motor deficit is due to this temporary inactivation of neuronal activity, rather than to the permanent destruction of a necessary part of the neural substrate for a given type of movement, the potential to carry out that type of movement should return as the shock state diminishes. However, the nature of the learned nonuse mechanism is such that it will supervene whenever a serious motor deficit is present. Subsequently, the learned nonuse mechanism will operate to suppress the return of movement potentially made possible by the recovery from CNS shock.

Since the mechanism operates in terms of the conditions of punishment and reward of attempted motor activity that pertain whenever CNS damage gives rise to a motor deficit, it should operate whatever the location of the nervous system injury that produces the deficit. Moreover, if two motor deficits that have different anatomic origins are overtly similar in the nature of the movement affected and are both associated with the CNS shock/learned nonuse mechanism, it is not unreasonable to hypothesize that the process by which the two can be overcome is similar.

The validity of this analysis can be evaluated empirically. If two deficits that are similar in nature but different in anatomic origin can be overcome by the same techniques, it follows from that analysis that one would have suggestive evidence that the same mechanism is involved in their remediation. It would still be conceivable that the resemblance was just phenotypic and that different mechanisms were involved in the two cases. However, the more parsimonious explanation would be that the same mechanism was involved in each case, especially if there was a strong conceptual basis for believing this to be true.

Research with Human Patients After Stroke

Preliminary application of one of the conditioned-response paradigms developed in primate deafferentation research to human stroke patients had taken place previously with some success (8,9). Subsequently, Wolf and co-workers (6,7) took the limb-restriction portion of the published protocol (but not the training component) and applied it to chronic stroke and traumatic brain injury patients. The results were promising. They stimulated the next research effort (13), which made modifications in the research design and added a training aspect (14) to the treatment of patients.

The subjects were chronic stroke patients who had experienced CVAs from one to eighteen years earlier. According to the traditional belief of the field, patients with this degree of chronicity have presumably reached a plateau in their motor recovery and will not exhibit any further improvement for the rest of their lives. The focal criterion for inclusion in the study was the ability to extend against gravity at least 20° at the wrist and 10° at the fingers. This criterion is derived empirically from work in which it showed a good correlation with the amount of recovery of motor recovery that occurred with another intervention following stroke. Approximately 20–25% of the chronic stroke population with motor deficit are capable of meeting or exceeding this requirement (40), and are therefore presumably optimally amenable to the treatment approach to be described.

Nine persons who met the study's inclusion criteria were assigned by a random process to either an experimental group (four subjects) or an attention-comparison group (five subjects). The subjects in the two groups were closely matched in initial motor ability and did not diverge significantly in major demographic characteristics or in chronicity (median 4.1 years for the restraint group; median 4.5 years for the comparison group).

For the experimental group, the unaffected limb was secured in a resting hand splint and placed in a sling; the affected arm was left free. The subjects agreed to wear the movement constraint device for approximately 90% of waking hours for twelve days. On each of the eight weekdays during this period, patients spent seven hours at the rehabilitation center and were given a variety of tasks to be carried out by the paretic upper extremity for six hours (e.g., eating lunch with a fork and spoon; throwing a ball; playing dominoes, Chinese checkers, or card games; writing on paper or on a chalkboard; pushing a broom; using the Purdue Dexterity Board; taking the Minnesota Rate of Manipulation Test). No explicit training of any kind, including shaping, was given; the subjects simply practiced the tasks repeatedly. The purpose was primarily to provide experience in use of the affected limb.

The procedures given to the comparison group were designed to focus attention on the involved extremity. This was accomplished in three ways. First, patients were told (during four periods on separate days) that they had much greater motor ability with their affected extremity than they were exhibiting; they were exhorted to focus attention at home on using the affected extremity in as many new activities as possible. Examples were given, and record keeping was required and monitored. Second, patients received two sessions (labeled physical therapy) involving only those activities that required neither active movement nor limbering of the involved limb. Third, patients were given self-range-of-movement exercises to carry out at home for fifteen minutes a day. In these exercises, the affected extremity was passively moved into a variety of positions by the unaffected extremity.

Two laboratory tests of motor function were administered to experimental and comparison subjects just before and immediately after their two-week intervention period. One test consisted of simple limb movements, half without functional end points (6). The other was composed of more complex tasks involving complete activities of daily living (41). To summarize the findings, there were significant changes in the motor ability of the subjects whose uninvolved extremity was restricted, and these changes were large. The mean performance time of the experimental subjects decreased 38% on the first test and 28% on the second (Figure 13-3). The subjects also exhibited substantial increases in measures of quality of movement and functional ability in

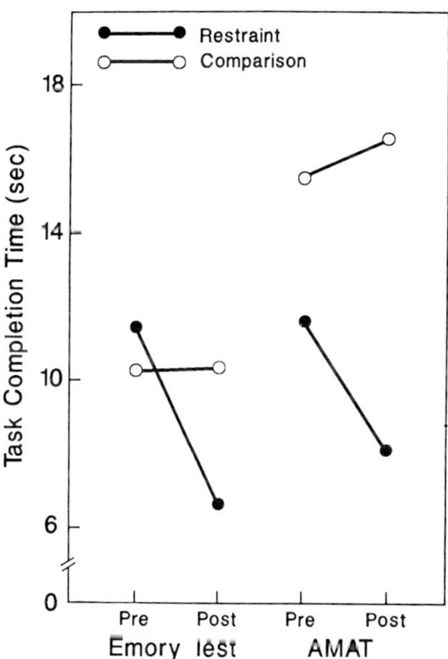

Figure 13-3. Mean task completion time (seconds) on two motor ability tests.

the two tests (Figure 13-4). In contrast, the performance of the comparison group was not significantly changed at their postintervention testing on any of these parameters.

A third instrument, the Motor Activity Log (MAL), provided information about motor function in the normal environment, thus addressing the critical issue of generalization. This log consists of ratings of fourteen common and important activities of daily life from such functional areas as feeding, dressing, and grooming. The comparison subjects did not improve on this scale in relation to the year preceding their entry into the project. In contrast, the movement-restriction subjects improved almost 2.5 rating steps (out of six) (Figure 13-5). There was virtually no overlap in the records of the two groups during treatment or during the follow-up period (Figure 13-6). Moreover, the treatment gains of the experimental subjects were fully maintained two years after the completion of the two weeks of treatment. Thus, the increase in the amount of use of the limb was long-term and quite possibly permanent.

The improvement of the movement-restriction patients in MAL scores in part reflects better quality of movement and in part reflects the fact that these patients were able to translate the improvements made in the laboratory into mastery of a large range of daily activities that they had not previously carried out with the affected arm. The new activities included brushing teeth, combing hair, picking up a glass of water and drinking, eating with a fork or spoon, and writing, among others. There was a

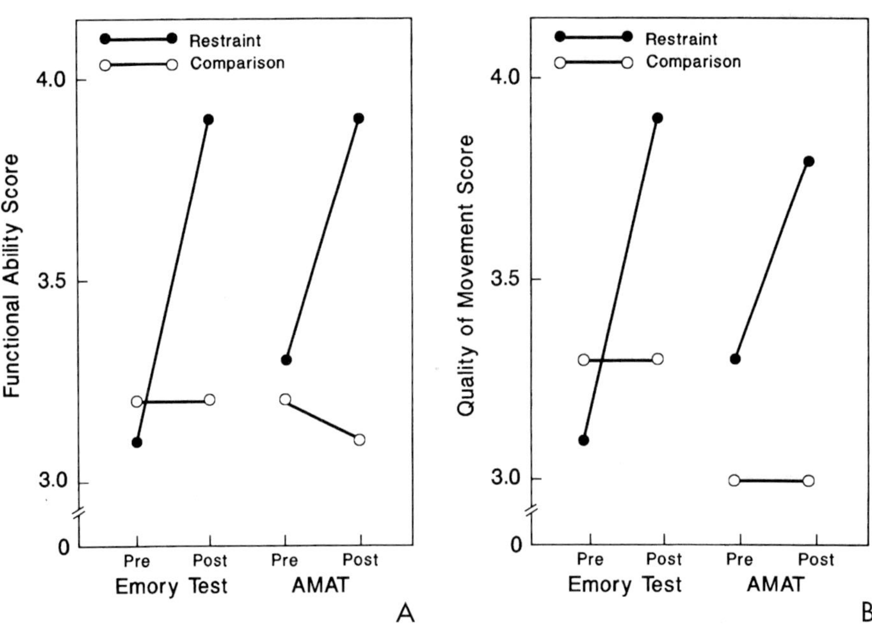

Figure 13-4. Mean functional ability (A) and quality of movement (B) on two motor ability tests.

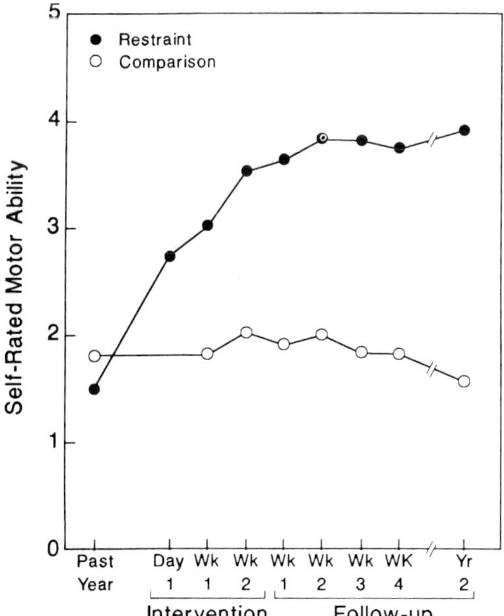

Figure 13-5. Group data on Motor Activity Logs.

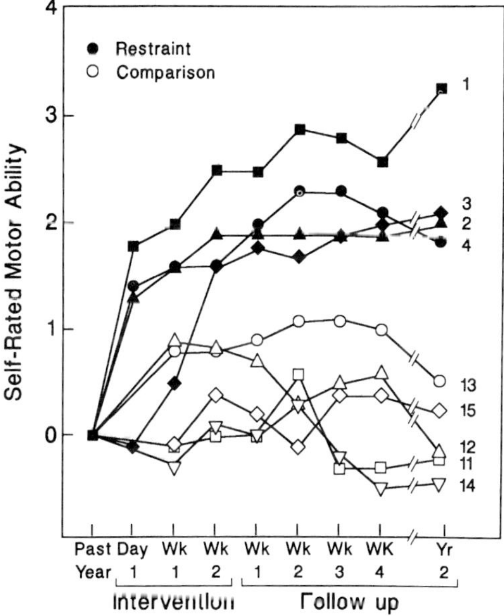

Figure 13-6. Individual data on Motor Activity Logs. The data are ipsitized so that each subject's pretreatment score is set to zero.

mean increase of 97.1% in the number of activities on the MAL that the patients reported they could carry out one month after restraint compared to the period before treatment. The comparable change for the comparison subjects was 14.5%. The difference between groups on this measure was statistically significant after the interventions (U test, p < .01), but not before.

In interviews, the restraint patients stated that they were capable of a greatly expanded range of activities. They reported that they had made major gains in what was, in effect, functional independence. This is consistent with the results from the MAL. In the most dramatic case, motor improvement was great enough to permit part-time clerical employment. One of this subject's main tasks was answering the phone with the unaffected hand and writing messages with the affected hand. She was thus able to relieve a self-reported depressed state because she previously "had nothing to do except spend most of my days staring at the four walls of my apartment." A second, more recent subject has also resumed employment.

▨▨▨ *Recent Research with Human Stroke Patients*

Since publication of this research, work has been completed with thirteen additional subjects using three different modified treatment protocols. Investigators who contributed importantly to this research were Drs. Donna M. Bearden, Jay M. Meythaler, Louis D. Burgio, and Stacey Goode. The recent work was carried out in the same experimental room as the earlier work, with the same equipment (where appropriate), the same pre- and post-treatment test battery, and the participation of the current co-authors (ET and JEC), who also worked on the first experiment and communicated the project's procedures to its new collaborators. It would, therefore, seem legitimate to consider the results from the two groups described in the published article as the beginning of a long-term study that continues with the recent work to be described below. There would thus be five groups. Groups 1 and 2 would be the experimental and control groups from the published article, respectively, while Groups 3–5 would include the subjects from the recent research. A brief description of the treatment procedure employed in each group follows.

> *Group 1*—Sling restraint of the unaffected upper extremity and supervised task practice with the affected arm (but no explicit training)—four subjects.
> *Group 2*—Attention control procedures—five subjects.
> *Group 3*—Sling restraint of the unaffected arm plus shaping of movements of the affected arm—five subjects.
> *Group 4*—Half-glove on the unaffected hand as a reminder not to use it plus shaping of movements of the affected arm—four subjects.
> *Group 5*—Shaping of movements of the affected arm only (no constraint of unaffected arm movement)—four subjects.

The results from the recent work (Groups 3–5) are currently being analyzed statistically, and at the date of this writing the analysis has not been completed. Given the many dependent measures that are used to evaluate the effects of the interventions (13) and the small sample size, consideration of only group means without any indication of which differences are significant might yield a false impression. Consequently, at this time the most appropriate course would be to provide a general evaluation of the treatment results based on close inspection of the data during the data ordering and data entry process. It is unlikely that the statistical results will importantly alter the conclusions arrived at in this fashion.

Group 3—Sling Restraint Plus Shaping

As noted previously, shaping is a widely used behavioral training technique in which a desired motor or behavioral objective is approached in small steps, by successive approximations (27–31). The technique has been used extensively with adults with mental retardation, self-injurious behavior, elderly persons exhibiting inactivity or disruptive behavior, motor deficits, children with autism, and children with behavioral problems, as well as a variety of other conditions. Shaping is very similar to the procedure engaged in by physical therapists and occupational therapists when giving patients task practice. The primary difference lies in the emphasis given in shaping to explicit verbal feedback concerning small changes in performance and the small steps into which planned progress is divided. Essentially, it is primarily an explication and formalization of procedures already in use in the field of physical rehabilitation.

At the beginning of work with a subject in this experiment, new tasks are often designed that are tailored to provide training for the movements that are most impaired in that individual. Each task must have aspects that are easily quantifiable, preferably so that small improvements are immediately apparent to the subject. Rest intervals are introduced in each shaping session. The rest periods are usually the same length as the trial periods, although longer intervals are sometimes used to prevent fatigue. Verbal reinforcement is given enthusiastically after the smallest performance improvements are detectable. The experimenter's verbal response is intended to provide detailed information in terms of the specific nature of the improvements. Additionally, maintenance of previous gains is acknowledged on each occasion. Performance regressions are never punished and are usually ignored. When performance has not increased for approximately three trials, the subject is encouraged to improve further (e.g., "Let's see whether we can do a little more on the next try"). Liberal use is made of modeling and prompts. At the beginning of a shaping series, subjects may be given physical help in carrying out parts of a movement sequence they cannot do themselves. In physical therapy, this is termed *assisted movement*. This aid is attenuated and then faded out as soon as is feasible. If a subject is having too much trouble making progress in a task, a simpler task involving similar movements is substituted.

In preliminary work with practice subjects, a battery of approximately thirty tasks was developed with a preliminary shaping plan for each (42). Since different individuals have different levels of motor function and response to therapy, the shaping plan is adapted to each individual. The actual subset of tasks selected for use with each subject depends on such factors as (1) specific joint movements that exhibit the most pronounced deficit, (2) the joint movements that project staff believe have the greatest potential for improvement, (3) subject preference among tasks that have a similar potential for producing specific improvements.

In our research with deafferented monkeys, shaping stood partway between our earlier conditioned-response training procedures and device restriction of movement of the intact limb, both conceptually and empirically, in its ability to enable generalization from the experimental situation to the natural environment. Although shaping and intact-limb restriction superficially represent two different approaches to the rehabilitation of movement (but see last section), they are not mutually exclusive; indeed, from the outset they appeared to be potentially complementary. These two procedures were not employed jointly in the research with monkeys; however, it seemed reasonable to attempt this approach in work with human stroke patients. Some of the shaping tasks employed are listed here, but by name only, to provide a general idea of their nature. This list is not exhaustive: shuffleboard, rotate a Rolodex file, tap a telegraph key, shave (capped blade and simulated with formalized movements), ring placement on a peg-horizontal, ring placement on a peg-vertical, trace circles within printed inner and outer boundaries, brush teeth, open spring-loaded clothespins and clip them onto the wires of a cake rack, use wrench to screw bolts into threaded holes on a child's workbench, hammer plastic nails into holes, use screwdriver to turn screws, make dot-to-dot drawings, wash hands (simulated with formalized movements), dry hands (simulated with formalized movements), use children's building blocks to create a tall edifice, insert electrical plugs into a power strip, turn pages, place graduated weights on different height boxes, open flip-top shampoo bottle with thumb, depress lever 1/4 inch on plastic infant's toy until a light is illuminated, write signature, move children's wooden building blocks from location to location.

The results indicate that when shaping is added to sling restraint of the unaffected upper extremity, it does not confer any therapeutic advantage as compared to having just supervised task practice plus sling restraint in increasing ability to use the affected upper extremity in the life situation. Initially, we were surprised at this outcome. Although shaping had never been combined with intact limb restraint in deafferented monkeys, as noted above, shaping by itself had produced impressive results with these animals in the rehabilitation of movement. It was therefore intuitively thought that the robust results obtained with these two techniques when used individually would add together, at least partially, when they were used together. It was expected that this would lead to a better result in chronic stroke patients than that obtained with supervised practice combined with restraint. In retrospect, however, reasons why the addition of shaping might not lead to a further increment in motor ability become obvious. First, the combination of unaffected limb restraint and supervised practice over a two-week period led to so good a result in Group 1 that one might reasonably have expected that a ceiling had been achieved. The mean post-treatment score of Group 1 experimental subjects on the Motor Activity Log, which takes data on the amount of use of the affected upper extremity in the life situation, was "4," a score whose anchoring definition is "almost normal." Since these subjects had sustained substantial brain damage as a result of their CVAs, an amount of affected limb use that is "almost normal" could well be the physiological maximum that their neurological status permitted. No treatment, no matter how effective, could be expected to improve motor function beyond that ceiling. Second, supervised practice can be conceptualized as a type of shaping where the reinforcement is provided by the environment (that is, by the success or failure achieved in the tasks that the subjects attempt), rather than being provided by a therapist, as in shaping. Supervised practice might not be as effective in inducing post-stroke motor improvement in chronic patients as shaping, but in combination with unaffected upper extremity restraint it might be quite effective. Moreover, its relative efficacy in comparison to shaping is still very much an open question that must be resolved empirically.

If further research confirms that unaffected upper extremity restraint plus supervised practice is as effective a treatment as restraint plus shaping, this would have positive cost-effectiveness implications. Shaping is a time-intensive procedure that involves a one-on-one interaction with a therapist. In contrast, supervised task practice involves much less of the therapist's time and attention. Two and possibly three patients can be worked with simultaneously; they could, for example, be asked to engage in group activities with one another.

Group 4—Half-Glove Plus Shaping

The subjects in this group received shaping of movements of the affected upper extremity; but instead of receiving sling-restraint of the unaffected limb, they agreed to wear a half-glove on the unaffected hand for 90% of waking hours. The purpose of the glove was to serve as a reminder, every time the subject saw it, not to use the unaffected arm. The half-glove left the fingers free, was comfortable, and was jokingly referred to by project staff as the "magic glove." During the seven hours subjects spent with project staff each weekday, considerable time was devoted to focusing attention on the role of the glove and on getting subjects adapted to employing it as a cue to not use the unaffected upper extremity. Additionally, as with all other groups, the first half hour of each weekday morning was spent: (1) filling out the Motor Activity Log, and (2) going over a diary that subjects kept of their activities at home, including the times when the constraint device was worn, when it was not worn, and the activities that were carried out during these periods. For the half-glove subjects, this initial half-hour period was used to further emphasize the importance of using the glove for its intended purpose.

The results were again surprising. Improvement in quality of movement and amount of use of the affected upper extremity in activities of daily living in the life situation was just as great for the Group 4 half-glove subjects as for the Group 1 sling-restraint subjects. Thus, there appears to be nothing talismanic, as it were, about use of the sling. Any method for effectively focusing attention on not using the unaffected limb and promoting sustained use of the affected extremity would appear to accomplish a substantial rehabilitation of movement in chronic stroke patients meeting this project's minimum motor criterion.

The major advantage of using the half-glove is that it enables use of the overcoming learned nonuse approach with patients who have balance problems, or even with patients who spend all or part of the day in a wheelchair. If a patient were to fall while wearing a sling, the unaffected upper extremity could not be employed to break the descent. Thus, for safety reasons, balance problems were one of the exclusion criteria of this project. By being able to use a half-glove rather than a sling, our project has tripled the size of the chronic stroke population that can be worked with.

Group 5—Shaping Only

The subjects in this group received shaping of the movement of the affected limb on each weekday during the two-week intervention period, just as in Groups 3 and 4. However, they were not given a device to wear on the unaffected upper extremity to constrain use of that limb. These subjects were also asked to try to use the affected limb outside the treatment center, and a diary of this usage was kept and reviewed daily, as in Groups 3 and 4. However, considerably less emphasis was placed on this instruction than in the other groups during the course of the treatment day.

For this group, use of the limb improved not only in the clinic but also in the life situation. Improvement on the laboratory motor tests and in range of motion occurred, and on many measures (but not all) it was as great as in the three constraint groups (Groups 1, 3, and 4). However, inspection of the data suggests that transfer of the improvement to the life situation, while substantial, was not as great as in the constraint groups. Given the effectiveness of shaping in the research with deafferented monkeys, the improvement in the clinic and the transfer to the life situation were to be expected. Determination of whether the apparent lesser amount of transfer to the life situation, compared to the three constraint conditions, is significant awaits the results of the current statistical analysis.

Recommendations Concerning Patient Characteristics Appropriate for the Different Techniques

Sling vs. Half-Glove

Adherence in wearing the constraint device will almost certainly be a problem with a certain, possibly large, percentage of patients with regard to clinical use of devices to constrain the use of the unaffected upper extremity. In our project, we are aided by the fact that patients are under the direct observation of project staff for the substantial period they spend in the rehabilitation center. During this time, at least, we are sure that they are adherent. Additionally, as noted previously, we spend considerable time reviewing each patient's home diary, which describes the use or nonuse of the constraint device. If the device is being worn for an insufficient amount of time, project staff spend time problem-solving with the patient on how device use might be increased and how various tasks can be carried out while using it. Special attention is paid during discussions throughout the day to details that might reveal whether the patient is conveying an accurate account; apparent discrepancies are employed as a basis for further problem-solving and for obtaining additional adherence. Because of the adherence issue, we recommend use of sling restraint whenever possible. However, when it is not possible, as when a patient has balance problems or is confined to a wheelchair, the half-glove should be used and should give good results.

If a half-glove is to be used, it would be optimal to carry out the intervention on an inpatient basis so that adherence can be monitored. If a person is to be treated on an outpatient basis, it would be advantageous to bring that individual into the treatment center, daily if possible. (This is clearly also the case for sling-restraint patients.) If therapist time is not available for work with the patient for substantial blocks of time, or even if there is insufficient time to work with the patient at all, their presence in the treatment center would nevertheless promote adherence. In our current work (not reported here), we sometimes integrate project patients into the volunteer program of the rehabilitation center, where they carry out such routine tasks as putting out linens for the physical therapy work area, xeroxing, sorting mail, helping to transport patients, contacting inpatient family members, and so on. The loose supervision associated with these activities is helpful in increasing adherence.

Shaping vs. Supervised Practice

In our work, we continue to use shaping rather than supervised practice. However, one objective of some of our current research is to increase the sample size in the groups that we have already begun. For clinical purposes, it would probably be just as effective to use the less time-intensive supervised task practice, as long as it was employed in combination with constraint of the affected limb.

Home Practice

In all constraint groups (Groups 1, 3, and 4), we provide patients with an individually tailored home practice program consisting of twenty minutes of task practice and range of motion exercises that patients are asked to carry out daily. During follow-up, patients are questioned about and encouraged to do their home practice. An excellent model for home practice programs has been developed by Bach-y-Rita and co-workers (5).

Negative Results and Number of the Patients Potentially Amenable to This Form of Treatment

To date, one or another of the treatment protocols described above have been administered to nineteen chronic stroke patients, while five additional subjects were in an attention-control group. Eighteen of the nineteen treatment subjects reached or exceeded the project's minimum motor criterion of being capable of at least 20° extension at the wrist and 10° at the fingers. Seventeen of the eighteen subjects who met the project's minimum motor criterion completed their assigned protocol and were found to have improved substantially in amount of use of the affected limb; one of these eighteen subjects did not complete his protocol. Another individual was the sole person treated who did not meet the minimum motor criterion. The results of the latter two individuals are revealing and will be discussed below.

Early Terminating Subject

This 75-year-old male sustained a left-brain CVA fourteen months prior to entry into the project; he had been right dominant premorbidly. He was assigned to the Group 3 sling plus shaping procedure. Unknown to project staff, he had agreed to participate in the project only as a means of relief from the persistent demands of his spouse. An "expectancy" questionnaire, administered to each subject before the beginning of the intervention, revealed that he had no expectation that the project's procedures would have any effect on his ability to use the affected upper extremity, and this was amply confirmed verbally at a later time. After two days of unaffected limb restraint and shaping, project staff noted a typical marked increase in use of the affected extremity. However, the subject did not report perceiving an improvement in his motor status. On the third day, however, the patient did notice the large change in his motor ability and reported it accurately. On the fourth morning, he arrived at the project not wearing his sling; he presented it to staff members and announced that he was terminating his participation in the project. He explained that he had a second wife, who was twenty years younger than him, and twelve children, ten of whom lived near him. They took care of all his needs and he had to do very little for himself. This, he said, was the way he felt it should be after having spent his life working hard as a railroad employee. His unexpected motor improvement was jeopardizing his prized living arrangement, and he was therefore leaving the project before any more damage could be done. Although the subject did not betray any overt anger, he did refuse to participate in a one-hour motor testing session, to be held at that time at our urgent request.

While this case is amusing, it does point to the serious fact that people who are receiving secondary gains from their motor deficit cannot be expected to participate in or continue a treatment that is improving it. However, we have encountered this type of situation in only one of twenty-four subjects (nineteen experimental, five control). Most stroke patients are very strongly motivated to improve use of their affected extremities. We have also had good results with two subjects who exhibited mild to moderate depression scores on a depression scale with established reliability and validity for a stroke population (43). Apparently, patients who exhibit only mild to moderate depression still retain a strong desire to increase the ability to use their affected extremities.

Low Functioning Subject

We have worked with only one subject who did not meet the project's minimum motor criterion. This individual exhibited virtually no ability to extend wrist or fingers against gravity. He was given sling restraint and shaping (Group 3). While he did improve moderately during the course of shaping on some tasks, none of this improvement was translated into increased ability to carry out the activities of daily living. He is viewed as being the project's one treatment failure.

The percentage of patients who do not meet Wolf's informal criterion (40), which we have incorporated as this project's minimum motor requirement, but who would benefit from the constraint-induced facilitation therapeutic approach is at present unknown. If the one subject described in this section is an indication, it would clearly not be as high as with the experimental subjects worked with to date. However, at least some of these patients might also be helped. It is estimated that approximately 20–25% of chronic stroke patients with motor deficit can meet or exceed the project's minimum motor criterion without functioning at too high a level to make therapy irrelevant. Patients who have serious uncontrolled medical problems or who are excessively frail would not be good candidates for interventions involving one of the constraint-induced facilitation techniques. However, given the results from use of a half-glove, balance problems should not be a basis for exclusion. Reduced cognitive ability would exclude a patient from *experimental* work because confusion and inability to follow test instructions promptly would preclude the collection of meaningful quantitative data. However, reduced cognitive ability should not importantly reduce the value of constraint-induced facilitation techniques on a clinical basis. These techniques, after all, were first discovered in work with Macaque monkeys.

Excess Motor Disability: Extensions of the Constraint-Induced Facilitation Paradigm

Excess motor disability that is substantially greater than appears warranted by the organic condition of the individual is a common clinical observation. Its existence in any given case can often not be demonstrated conclusively, since by its nature it involves function that is not being expressed and can therefore not be observed. In this article we have described experiments indicating that following unilateral deafferentation in monkeys and stroke in humans there can be substantial excess motor disability that is maintained by a learned nonuse mechanism. However, it can be reversed. Similar results involving the use of techniques for overcoming learned nonuse following stroke have been obtained by Wolf and co-workers (6) and a number of other investigators (8–12). The extensive new motor function, which typically develops too rapidly for the learning of new motor skills to be involved, indicates that the motor ability being expressed had been latent, awaiting only the application of an appropriate therapeutic intervention. We have also cited evidence that excess motor disability can also occur following pyramidotomy and other motor lesions in monkeys (36–39). Of particular additional interest is the fact that Wolf and co-workers (6) have used a technique for overcoming learned nonuse in traumatic brain injury patients with predominantly unilateral motor involvement to substantially improve motor performance, thereby suggesting that the pretreatment deficit involved excess motor disability. Desai (12) has obtained similar results in clinical work.

Thus, learned nonuse may be a general mechanism and it may operate in a variety of conditions, not only after the neurological injuries just specified. The learned nonuse formulation indicates that any type of organic damage that results in an initial inability to carry out a function establishes the conditions of reward and punishment conducive to the development of learned nonuse; the operation of this mechanism becomes superimposed upon and strengthens the organically determined inability to carry out the function. If the anatomical or biochemical substrate whose impairment led to the initial deficit recovers or heals, learned nonuse could still hold recovery of function in check unless it is overcome. Until now the application of the learned nonuse mechanism has been studied only with respect to neurological impairment of an upper extremity. However, according to the formulation, the mechanism could also apply to other types of function such as speech (as in aphasia); other portions of the body, such as a lower extremity; or nonneural injury, such as skeletal system damage, e.g., after fractured hip. For these cases that portion of the deficit due to learned nonuse would be reversible by the application of an appropriate technique. This approach has been used recently by Birbaumer and Taub (unpublished data) for the successful rehabilitation of ambulation following spinal cord injury and for the treatment of pain-induced nonuse of a child's upper extremity (K. Burgio and Taub, unpublished data), both in single cases.

Naming the Intervention Paradigm: "Constraint-Induced Facilitation"

The sling-restraint of the unaffected arm employed in Groups 1 and 3 and in the work of Wolf and co-workers (6,7) could appropriately be referred to as involving a "forced use" paradigm (6). However, the supervised task practice in Group 1, the shaping employed in Groups 3–5, and the half-glove used in Group 4 have also been found to be effective in treatment, and they are not best described as involving "forced use." All of these interventions share one common feature; they all involve "constraint" of the movements of the unaffected limb. For the sling procedure, the constraint is physical. For the half-glove procedure, the constraint is in the form of a reminder during 90% of working hours not to use the affected limb. In a training situation, the subjects are constrained either to use the affected limb (and not the unaffected limb) or fail at their task. The unsupervised practice of Group 1 involves elements of the latter implicitly. A term that covers the commonality of all of these procedures is *constraint-induced facilitation* of impaired movement.

Acknowledgments: Supported by grants from the Veterans Administration (Rehab R & D Project B93-629 AP), The Retirement Research Foundation, and The Center from Aging, University of Alabama at Birmingham. We thank Hugh S. Gainer, Administrator and Samuel L. Stover, former director, Spain Rehabilitation Center, University of Alabama at Birmingham, for their help in implementing the study.

References

1. Franz SI, Scheetz ME, Wilson AA. The possibility of recovery of motor functioning in long-standing hemiplegia. *JAMA* 1915;65:2150–54.
2. Balliet R, Levy B, Blood KMT. Upper extremity sensory feedback therapy in chronic cerebrovascular accident patients with impaired expressive aphasia and auditory comprehension. *Arch Phys Med Rehabil* 1986;61:304–10.
3. Bach-y-Rita P. Recovery from brain damage. *J Neuro Rehab* 1993;6:191–99.
4. Bach-y-Rita P, Wicab Bach-y-Rita E. Biological and psychosocial factors in recovery from brain damage in humans. *Can J Psychol* 1990;44:148–65.
5. Bach-y-Rita P, McGinn M, Anderson D, Roszkowski J, Parent J. Late rehabilitation following brain injury: the NMRC experience. In: Simkins CN (ed.). *Analysis, understanding and presentation of cases involving traumatic brain injury.* Washington, D.C.: National Head Injury Foundation, 1994:191–98.
6. Wolf SL, Lecraw DE, Barton LA, Jann BB. Forced use of hemiplegic upper extremities to reverse the effect of learned nonuse among chronic stroke and head-injured patients. *Exp Neurol* 1989;104:104–32.
7. Ostendorf CG, Wolf SL. Effect of forced use of the upper extremity of a hemiplegic patient on changes in function. *J Am Phys Ther Assoc* 1981;61:1022–28.
8. Ince LP. Escape and avoidance conditioning of response in the plegic arm of stroke patients: a preliminary study. *Psychonom Sci* 1969;16:49–50.
9. Halberstam JL, Zaretsky HH, Brucker BS, Guttman A. Avoidance conditioning of motor responses in elderly brain-damaged patients. *Arch Phys Med Rehabil* 1971;52:318–28.

10. Tries JM. Learned nonuse: a factor in incontinence. In: Miller NE (Chair). Overcoming learned nonuse and the release of covert behavior as a new approach to physical medicine. Symposium conducted at the meeting of the Association for Applied Psychophysiology and Biofeedback. Dallas, 1991.

11. Tries J. EMG biofeedback for the treatment of upper-extremity dysfunction: can it be effective? *Biofeedback and Self-Regulation* 1989;14:21–53.

12. Desai V. Report on functional utility score change in nine chronic stroke or closed head injury patients receiving a training program for overcoming learned nonuse as part of a multi-modality treatment program. In: Miller NE (Chair). Overcoming learned nonuse and the release of covert behavior as a new approach to physical medicine. Symposium conducted at the meeting of the Association for Applied Psychophysiology and Biofeedback, Dallas, 1991.

13. Taub E, Miller NE, Novak TA, et al. Technique to improve chronic motor deficit after stroke. *Arch Phys Med Rehabil* 1993;74:347–54.

14. Taub E. Somatosensory deafferentation research with monkeys: implications for rehabilitation medicine. In: Ince LP (ed.). *Behavioral psychology in rehabilitation medicine: clinical applications*. New York: Williams & Wilkins, 1980:371–401.

15. Taub E. Movement in nonhuman primates deprived of somatosensory feedback. *Exercise and Sports Sciences Reviews* (Vol. 4). Santa Barbara: Journal Publishing Affiliates, 1977:335–74.

16. Mott FW, Sherrington CS. Experiments upon the influence of sensory nerves upon movement and nutrition of the limbs. *Proc R Soc Lond* 1895;57:481–88.

17. Lassek AM. Inactivation of voluntary motor function following rhizotomy. *J Neuropath Exp Neurol* 1953;3:83–87.

18. Twitchell TE. Sensory factors in purposive movement. *J Neurophysiol* 1954;17:239–54.

19. Knapp HD, Taub E, Berman AJ. Movements in monkeys with deafferented forelimbs. *Exp Neurol* 1963;7:305–15.

20. Stein BM, Carpenter MW. Effects of dorsal rhizotomy upon subthalamic dyskinesia in the monkey. *Arch Neurol* 1965;13:567–83.

21. Knapp HD, Taub E, Berman AJ. Effect of deafferentation on a conditioned avoidance response. *Science* 1959;128:842–43.

22. Taub E, Bacon R, Berman AJ. The acquisition of a trace-conditioned avoidance response after deafferentation of the responding limb. *J Comp Physiol Psychol* 1965;58:275–79.

23. Taub E, Berman AJ. Avoidance conditioning in the absence of relevant proprioceptive and exteroceptive feedback. *J Comp Physiol Psychol* 1963;56:1012–16.

24. Taub E, Ellman SJ, Berman AJ. Deafferentation in monkeys: effect on a conditioned grasp response. *Science* 1966;151:593–94.

25. Wylie RM, Tyner CF. Weight-lifting by normal and deafferented monkeys: evidence for compensatory changes in ongoing movements. *Brain Res* 1981;219:172–77.

26. Wylie RM, Tyner CF. Performance of a weight-lifting task by normal and deafferented monkeys. *Behav Neurosci* 1989;108:273–82.

27. Morgan WG. The shaping game: a teaching technique. *Behav Ther* 1974;5:271–72.

28. Risley TR, Baer DM. Operant behavior modification: the deliberate development of behavior. In: Caldwell M, Riciuti HN (eds.). *Review of child development research. Vol. III, Development and social action*. Chicago: University of Chicago Press, 1973.

29. Skinner BF. *The behavior of organisms*. New York: Appleton-Century-Crofts, 1938.

30. Skinner BF. *The technology of teaching*. New York: Appleton-Century-Crofts, 1968.

31. Panyan MV. *How to use shaping*. Lawrence, KS: H & H Enterprises, 1980.

32. Taub E, Goldberg IA, Taub PB. Deafferentation in monkeys: pointing at a target without visual feedback. *Exp Neurol* 1975;46:178–86.

33. Taub E, Perrella PN, Barro G. Behavioral development following forelimb deafferentation on day of birth in monkeys with and without blinding. *Science* 1973;181:959–60.

34. Taub E, Perrella PN, Miller EA, Barro G. Diminution of early environmental control through perinatal and prenatal somatosensory deafferentation. *Biol Psychiat* 1975;10:609–26.

35. Taub E, Berman AJ. Movement and learning in the absence of sensory feedback. In: Freedman SJ (ed.). *The neuropsychology of spatially oriented behavior.* Homewood, IL: Dorsey Press, 1968:173–92.

36. Ogden R, Franz SI. On cerebral motor control: the recovery from experimentally produced hemiplegia. *Psychobiol* 1917;1:33–47.

37. Tower SS. Pyramidal lesions in the monkey. *Brain* 1940;63:36–90.

38. Lashley KS. Studies of cerebral function in learning: V. the retention of motor areas in primates. *Arch Neurol Psychiat* 1924;12:249–76.

39. Chambers WW, Konorski J, Liu CN, Yu J, Anderson R. The effects of cerebellar lesions upon skilled movements and instrumental conditioned reflexes. *Acta Neurobiol Exp* 1972;32:721–32.

40. Wolf SL, Binder-Macleod SA. Electromyographic biofeedback applications to the hemiplegic patient: changes in upper extremity neuromuscular and functional status. *Phys Ther* 1983;63:1393–1403.

41. McCulloch K, Cook EW III, Fleming WC, Novack TA, Nepomuceno CS, Taub E. A reliable test of upper extremity ADL function. *Arch Phys Med Rehabil* 1988;67:755.

42. Taub E, Crago JE, Burgio LD, Groomes TE, Cook EW III, DeLuca S, Miller NE. An operant approach to rehabilitation medicine: overcoming learned nonuse by shaping. *J Exp Anal Behav* 1994;61:281–93.

43. Zung WWK. A self-rating depression scale. *Arch Gen Psychiat* 1965;12:63–70.

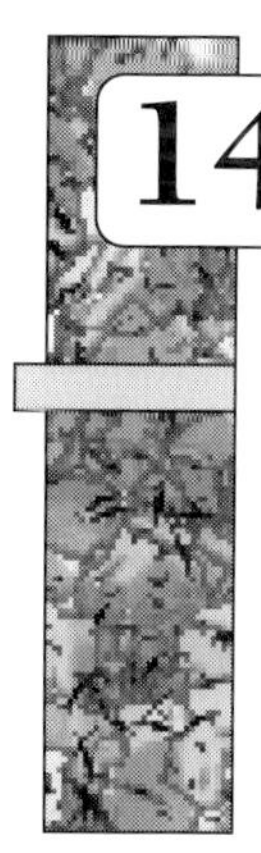

14

Pharmacologic Interventions for Improving Functional Tasks and Altering Brain Behavior

Larry B. Goldstein, M.D.

Introduction

Enhancement of functional recovery is one of the major goals of treatment after the acute phase of stroke. Facilitation of motor recovery is particularly important because motor function is one of the major determinants of independence in activities of daily living (1). Advances in the neurosciences over the last decade indicate that drugs influencing the activity of specific central neurotransmitters can modulate the recovery process. These drug effects may be either beneficial or harmful. Further, the drug effects may vary with the location of the lesion and with the target behavior. Based on these fundamental studies, a rudimentary clinical literature is developing concerning potential drug effects on recovery after stroke in humans (Table 14-1). These data not only suggest that pharmacotherapy to enhance recovery of lost function may be possible in selected patients, but as with experimental animal models, that some commonly prescribed medications used for the treatment of coincidental medical conditions may be harmful. New neuroimaging technologies may prove important in helping to determine which stroke patients may benefit from specific pharmacologic interventions and are providing insights into the mechanisms underlying the recovery process.

Experimental Studies

Sympathomimetic Amines and Related Drugs

Amphetamine is the prototypic catecholaminergic agonist with the capacity to enhance behavioral recovery after focal brain injury. Feeney and co-workers found that the administration of a single dose of d-amphetamine the day following a unilateral sensorimotor cortex injury in the rat resulted in an enduring enhancement of recovery (2). Post-lesion treatment with amphetamine also enhanced motor recovery in cats that had unilateral or bilateral frontal cortex ablations (3–5) and reinstated stereoscopic vision

Table 14-1. *Comparisons of the effects of various neurotransmitters and drugs on recovery following sensorimotor cortex injury with their effects on the induction of long-term potentiation (LTP).*

Transmitter/Drug	Effect on Recovery	Effect on LTP Induction
Norepinephrine	+	+
Amphetamine	+	+
Clonidine	−	−
Haloperidol	−	−
Prazosin	−	
Propranolol	Neutral	−
GABA	−	−
Diazepam	−	−
Muscimol	−	−
Phenytoin	−	
Acetylcholine	+	+
Scopolamine	−	−
MK-801	−/neutral	−

+ = a beneficial effect on recovery and a facilitation of the induction of LTP.
− = a detrimental effect on recovery and a suppression of the induction of LTP.
References are provided in the text.
Revised from Goldstein (8).

in cats with bilateral visual cortex lesions (6,7). Other laboratories have replicated the amphetamine effect, suggesting that it is quite robust (8,9). Amphetamine-facilitated recovery is also found after experimental focal traumatic (10) and ischemic (11) lesions. However, amphetamine administration was ineffective in promoting cognitive recovery after transient forebrain ischemia in gerbils, suggesting that the effect may not generalize to more diffuse central lesions or to all behaviors (12). Importantly, the beneficial behavioral effect of amphetamine is greatly diminished if rats are not given task-relevant experience in conjunction with the administration of the drug (2,6,7,13). These data indicate a synergistic effect between the drug and behavioral experience and suggest that amphetamine might act by facilitating a "relearning" process. Although amphetamine may influence the release of a variety of neurotransmitters, its effect on recovery is hypothesized to be related to enhanced release of central norepinephrine (14). Supporting this hypothesis, the impact on recovery of other adrenergic agonists and antagonists can be predicted based on their effects on the release of norepinephrine from noradrenergic terminals.

Other sympathomimetic agents studied in the laboratory include *phentermine*, an amphetamine analog with weaker cardiovascular effects, which accelerated motor recovery in both rats and cats (15). *Phenylpropanolamine*, at high doses, also facilitated recovery (16,17). However, the administration of a single dose of *methylphenidate*, a piperidine derivative structurally similar to amphetamine, had only a transient beneficial effect on locomotor function after sensorimotor cortex injury in rats (18). The lack of effectiveness of methylphenidate may be due to its short half-life. Repeated dosing of the drug has not been studied. Although not sympathomimetic amines, both *yohimbine* and *idazoxan* (centrally acting α_2-adrenergic receptor antagonists) increased norepinephrine release and enhanced motor recovery when given as a single dose after unilateral sensorimotor injury in rats (19–22).

Antihypertensives

Centrally acting α_2-adrenergic receptor antagonists enhance recovery in the rat hemiplegia model. Therefore, it is not surprising that a centrally acting α_2-adrenergic receptor agonist which diminishes norepinephrine release would be deleterious. *Clonidine,* when given even as a single dose the day after cortex injury, had a prolonged detrimental effect on motor recovery in rats (23). When given to rats that had recovered motor function, the administration of clonidine reinstated the motor deficit (22,24). *Prazosin* (22,25) and *phenoxybenzamine* (25,26), centrally acting α_2-adrenergic receptor antagonists, are also harmful. *Propranolol,* a nonselective β-adrenergic receptor antagonist, had no effect on motor recovery in animal models of motor recovery after focal cortical injury (25).

Major Tranquilizers

Coadministration of the butyrophenone *haloperidol* blocked amphetamine-promoted motor recovery in rats and haloperidol impaired motor recovery when given alone (2). When given to rats that had recovered, haloperidol as well as other butyrophenones (*fluanisone, droperidol*) transiently reinstated the motor deficit (27). Haloperidol administration also blocked amphetamine-facilitated recovery of stereopsis in visually decorticated cats (7,28). Although haloperidol is a dopamine receptor antagonist, it has antagonist effects at noradrenergic receptors (29–31). The available pharmacologic data suggest that the detrimental effect of haloperidol is mediated noradrenergically rather than through a dopaminergic mechanism. Intraventricular administration of dopamine had a nonsignificant beneficial effect on recovery from hemiplegia after sensorimotor cortex injury in rats (32). If a dopamine-β-hydroxylase inhibitor (blocking the conversion of dopamine to norepinephrine) was given in conjunction with intraventricular dopamine, the weak beneficial effect was blocked.

Tricyclic Antidepressants

As a class, the tricyclic antidepressants may affect a variety of neurotransmitters including norepinephrine, serotonin, and dopamine. Specific agents may have a greater or lesser selectivity for a specific neurotransmitter system. Several studies have been performed to examine the effects of these agents on behavioral recovery. The administration of a single dose of *trazodone* transiently slowed motor recovery in rats with sensorimotor cortex injury and reinstated the hemiparesis in recovered animals (33). In contrast, when rats were given a single dose of *desipramine,* a facilitation of motor recovery was observed (33). Although desipramine acts by inhibiting the reuptake of norepinephrine, it causes a decrease in the firing of presynaptic noradrenergic neurons through a feedback mechanism (34,35). Repeated administration of desipramine actually reduced brain norepinephrine content (36). Therefore, the effects of repeated dosing of the drug on recovery may be different from that seen after the administration of a single dose. The varying effects of single and repeated administration of these drugs is important when considering their potential effects on recovery in humans.

Anxiolytics

The prior sections have focused on catecholaminergic drugs and their impact on the recovery process. However, catecholamines are not the sole class of central neurotransmitters that may influence recovery after injury to the cerebral cortex. γ-aminobutyric acid (GABA) is one of the major inhibitory central neurotransmitters. The potential deleterious effect of drugs that enhance the action of GABA was suggested by a study that found the hemiparesis produced by a small motor cortex lesion in rats was increased by local GABA infusion (37). Benzodiazepines act as indirect GABA agonists and would be anticipated to be harmful if given during the recovery process. In fact, the short-term administration of *diazepam* permanently impeded recovery from the sensory asymmetry caused by anteromedial neocortex damage in the rat (38–40). The long-term deleterious effect of diazepam was mimicked by short-term infusion of the GABA agonist *muscimol* into the sensorimotor cortex adjacent to the lesion (41) and was blocked by coadministration of the benzodiazepine antagonist *Ro 15-1788* (41). Ro 15-1788 alone produced a transient facilitation of recovery (43). Anxiolytics that do not act through the GABA/benzodiazepine receptor complex may not interfere with recovery (43). *Gepirone* is an anxiolytic with no activity at the benzodiazepine receptor. Chronic administration of this drug did not impair recovery from the sensory asymmetry caused by anteromedial neocortex injury in the rat. Thus, this class of drugs may provide an alternative to benzodiazepines in patients recovering from stroke who require treatment with an anxiolytic.

Anticonvulsants

In addition to their anxiolytic effects, benzodiazepines are also potent anticonvulsants. The deleterious effect of GABA on motor recovery after cortex injury was increased by the systemic administration of *phenytoin* (44), which may act through a GABA-mediated mechanism (45). *Phenobarbital* also delayed behavioral recovery after injury to the cerebral cortex in laboratory studies (46,47). In contrast, chronic administration of *carbamazepine* in anticonvulsant doses did not affect sensory recovery after anteromedial cortex injury in rats (48). *MK-801* is a noncompetitive N-methyl-D-aspartate (NMDA) receptor antagonist with anticonvulsant activity that has been under intense study as a neuroprotective agent. The administration of MK-801 had no effect on motor recovery in the rat hemiplegia model (49), no effect on recovery of limb placing, and facilitated recovery of the sensory asymmetry resulting from anteromedial cortex injury (50). The drug had no effect on sensory function but reinstated forelimb placing deficits in rats that had recovered from anteromedial cortex injury (50). Thus, not all anticonvulsants have the same profile with regard to their impact on recovery. As with amphetamine, individual agents may have differing effects depending on the location of the lesion and the behavior being measured.

Anticholinergics

In 1942 Ward and Kennard reported that cholinergic agonists increased the rate of motor recovery after motor cortex lesions in monkeys (51). More recent data suggest that the anticholinergic drug *scopolamine* interfered with motor recovery following cortex infarction in rats (52). However, scopolamine treatment improved recovery following both concussive head injury (53) and unilateral ablation of the sensorimotor cortex (54) in rats. Thus, the experimental data concerning the impact of cholinergic drugs on recovery after brain injury are conflicting, and as with the amphetamine and the anticonvulsants, may vary according to the location of the lesion, the mechanism of injury, and the behaviors being measured.

Mechanisms

The mechanisms underlying spontaneous behavioral recovery after focal brain injury are likely varied and undoubtedly complex. Recovery may partially be due to resolution of some of the pathologic sequelae of acute brain injury. Additional potential active mechanisms of recovery have been divided into two general groups: rapidly developing physiologic responses and more slowly developing adaptive responses. There may be considerable overlap between these major classes of mechanisms. Each of the potential mechanisms may be influenced by drugs that affect the action of central neurotransmitters.

Relearning

Both laboratory and clinical evidence point to the importance of extrinsic environmental factors to the recovery process. For example, with regard to motor deficits, rats reared in enriched environments show less severe deficits after motor cortex lesions than controls housed in standard laboratory cages (55). Furthermore, task-specific post-lesion training alone is quite effective in enhancing motor recovery (56–58). As discussed previously, experience is required for both the positive and detrimental effects of catecholaminergic agents. Because motor recovery is so strongly influenced by environmental factors, one hypothesis is that the recovery entails a type of relearning.

The best understood cellular mechanism of learning and memory is long-term potentiation (LTP) (59–61). In the hippocampal formation, LTP is induced by a single, transient, high-frequency stimulation of excitatory neural inputs. This produces an increase in synaptic responses that can last for prolonged periods of time (60,61). LTP has been demonstrated in several other brain regions including hypothalamus (61), visual cortex (63,64), and motor cortex (65). If a relearning mechanism underlies recovery, then drugs that facilitate the induction of LTP would be expected to be beneficial whereas those that impair the induction of LTP would be detrimental. The available experimental data suggest that predictions based on this assumption are true for many, but not all, drugs.

Unmasking

Unmasking implies redundant neural pathways that "take over" for damaged ones. Positron emission tomography studies in human stroke patients show metabolic changes consistent with this phenomenon (66). In uninjured humans, motor movement is associated with increases in regional cerebral blood flow (rCBF) in a circumscribed region in the contralateral primary sensorimotor cortex. However, in patients recovered from stroke that had resulted in limb paresis, movement of the previously affected extremity is associated with significant changes in rCBF in widespread areas of the brain including both ipsilateral and contralateral sensorimotor cortex and cerebellar hemispheres (67–69). In that this phenomenon may be influenced by environmental factors, it may also entail a type of relearning, albeit through a mechanism different from that described in the preceding section.

Diaschisis

Diaschisis refers to a depression on neural function in structures that are remote from the site of primary injury and has been demonstrated experimentally in a variety of laboratory animal models (70–74). The potential effects of certain drugs on diaschisis form the basis of an attractive hypothesis for considering their effects on recovery after focal cortical injury (75). In human stroke patients, diaschisis-like changes in metabolism have been demonstrated by positron emission tomography in the noninjured ipsilateral cerebral hemisphere, the contralateral cerebral hemisphere, and the contralateral cerebellum (76–79). Crossed cerebellar-cortical diaschisis occurs in patients with unilateral cerebellar infarction (80). Deep hemispheric strokes can have remote effects on metabolism in both the cerebral cortex and cerebellum (81). Drugs that promote the resolution of diaschisis would be anticipated to facilitate recovery whereas those that prolong or worsen diaschisis would be anticipated to be detrimental. However, a clinical correlate of diaschisis and its resolution are currently lacking.

Neuronal Rearrangements

The slow adaptive responses involve anatomic neuronal rearrangements that occur after many types of brain injuries. Some of these neuronal reorganizations would be expected to be beneficial while others are potentially maladaptive (82). For a drug (such as a ganglioside or growth factor) to enhance behavioral recovery by influencing these types of neuronal alterations, it would have to selectively facilitate the favorable rearrangements and/or retard potentially harmful ones. Alternatively, a drug could be harmful if it interferes with adaptive rearrangements or promotes maladaptive ones. For example, the administration of an NMDA receptor antagonist after unilateral injury to the forelimb sensorimotor cortex in rats blocks certain neuronal rearrangements and interferes with recovery of forelimb function (50). Drugs that influence other central neurotransmitters may also have direct neuronotrophic effects that could affect the recovery process [see (83) for review].

Drugs and Recovery in Humans

The use of drugs to improve recovery after brain injury in humans had been attempted as early as the 1940s. More recent preliminary clinical studies indicate that many of the same drugs that influence recovery in laboratory animals have similar effects on recovery in humans.

Amphetamine

Motivation in elderly patients refractory to rehabilitation procedures improves with amphetamine treatment (84). This effect is likely nonspecific and due to the stimulant effects of the drug. However, several other anecdotal reports and small controlled trials suggest that treatment with amphetamine may enhance functional recovery after focal brain injury under certain conditions.

A small, prospective, double-blind study was carried out to determine whether amphetamine-facilitated motor recovery occurs in humans after stroke (85). The study was carefully designed to stimulate the paradigm used in the laboratory experimental studies. A group of eight patients with stable motor deficits within ten days of ischemic stroke were randomized to receive either a single dose of amphetamine or placebo. Motor function was measured with a reliable and validated scale, the Fugl-Meyer Assessment (86). Within three hours of drug administration, all of the patients underwent intensive physical therapy (e.g., drug administration was coupled with task-specific experience). The following day, the patients' abilities to use their affected limbs were reassessed. Overall, the amphetamine-treated group had a significant improvement in motor performance while there was little change in the placebo-treated group. It should be noted that only two of the four amphetamine-treated patients had a "dramatic" motor improvement (the intervention had a variable effect even in this highly selected group). Further, because this study involved only a small group of highly selected patients, the results may not be applicable to stroke patients with other types of deficits. Because only short-term recovery was measured, the longer-term efficacy of amphetamine treatment is unknown.

Due to concern about the potential harmful effects of sympathomimetic agents in patients immediately following stroke, studies reproducing and extending this facility have been lacking. One preliminary double-blind, placebo-controlled study was designed to determine whether treatment with amphetamine would enhance motor recovery in stroke rehabilitation patients (87). Patients were treated with amphetamine or placebo daily for three weeks with a final assessment one week after the last day of drug administration. The difference between the amphetamine and placebo-treated groups was not statistically significant. However, treatment was delayed until the patients were transferred to a rehabilitation hospital and they did not receive physical therapy in tight conjunction with amphetamine administration, possibly limiting the potential benefit of the drug.

A second double-blind, placebo-controlled trial of the effect of amphetamine on motor recovery in the rehabilitation setting include five amphetamine-treated and five placebo-treated patients (88). Drug or placebo was given once every four days for ten sessions beginning fifteen to thirty days after stroke. Each dose was given in conjunction with a session of intensive physical therapy. Motor function was again measured with the Fugl-Meyer Assessment, with the final evaluation one week after the last dose. Patients treated with amphetamine had significantly greater improvements in motor scores compared to placebo-treated patients. Although preliminary, these results suggest that amphetamine may enhance motor recovery in human stroke patients when drug administration is combined with task-relevant experience.

Speech pathologists have been particularly interested in studying the effects of drugs on language recovery after stroke. Preliminary studies indicate that the administration of bromocriptine improves fluency in certain aphasics (89–91) and that treatment with amphetamine may accelerate recovery from aphasia in stroke patients (92). A feasibility study of the effects of amphetamine on language recovery after stroke was recently carried out (93). Six aphasic patients had language function rated with the Porch Index of Communicative Ability ten to thirty days after stroke. Based on this initial evaluation, six month language scores were predicted for each patient. All patients were then given 10 mg d-amphetamine followed by speech therapy every fourth day for ten sessions. The patients' actual scores at three months were then compared with their six month predicted scores. Most patients achieved or exceeded their six month predicted scores by the time of the three month evaluation. A randomized prospective trial is now planned.

Tricyclic Antidepressants

Clinical depression is associated with impaired recovery after stroke in humans (94). Tricyclic antidepressants are commonly used to treat mood disorders in stroke patients. Trazodone, a drug that impairs recovery from hemiplegia in the rat, was found to improve outcome as measured with the Barthel Index in depressed stroke patients (95). However, trazodone was given in only a single dose in the animal study and repeated dosing likely has a different effect of neurotransmitter levels. Therefore, recommendations concerning the choice of specific tricyclic antidepressants in stroke patients must await further laboratory and clinical studies.

Other Catecholaminergic Drugs

Phenoxybenzamine caused slight transient worsening of the neurologic deficit in several stroke patients, but this might be due to the hemodynamic effects of the drug (96). One retrospective study found that both thiazide diuretics and a mixed group of antihypertensives were associated with impaired language recovery in aphasic stroke patients (97). Propranolol, a drug that had no effect on motor recovery in experimental studies, also had no effect on language recovery in these patients.

The Use of Potentially Detrimental Drugs

Although the previous discussion has focused on the use of drugs to enhance recovery after stroke, it is important to recognize that the laboratory studies suggest that some drugs may be detrimental. We carried out a retrospective study of physician prescribing patterns to determine what drugs were used in the treatment of stroke patients (98). Over 80% of individuals were taking at least one drug at the time of the stroke. Sixty-five percent of patients were receiving multiple drugs. Antihypertensives such as clonidine and prazosin and sedative hypnotics including benzodiazepines were among the most commonly prescribed agents. Thus, several of the drugs that have deleterious effects on recovery of function in laboratory animals were commonly prescribed for stroke patients for the treatment of coincident medical conditions.

Determining whether the detrimental effects of drugs anticipated from laboratory studies also occur in humans recovering from stroke is difficult. Largely anecdotal reports indicate that treatment with haloperidol (17,99) and certain antihypertensives (97) may interfere with language recovery in patients with aphasia following stroke. We performed a retrospective study that tested the hypothesis that drugs that are harmful during recovery in laboratory animals would interfere with motor recovery in human stroke patients (100). These potentially deleterious drugs included the antihypertensives clonidine and prazosin, neuroleptics, benzodiazepines, and phenytoin. The motor recoveries of stroke patients who received one or a combination of these drugs were compared to the recoveries of a similar group of patients who were not given any of these agents. The two groups were similar with respect to a variety of characteristics including age, blood pressure, gender, and medical comorbidity. Motor function was measured prospectively with the Fugl-Meyer Assessment by observers who were blind to the study hypothesis. Although the results of this study need to be interpreted with caution, patients who received one or a combination of the hypothesized "detrimental" drugs at the time of stroke or during the subsequent hospitalization had significantly slower motor recoveries than a comparable group of patients who did not receive one of these drugs. A multivariate analysis indicated a significant effect of "drug group" after correcting for the contributions of other variables including the initial severity of the deficit. Supporting these findings, the deleterious effect of certain drugs on motor recovery was also found in a separate cohort of patients with anterior circulation ischemic stroke (101).

The Potential Role of Neuroimaging

Variability in individual responses to drugs is expected based on both experimental and the available clinical data. The factors underlying this variability are only partially understood. Information that may partially explain this variability include differing lesion locations, pathologic sequelae of injury, and capacity for rapid or more slowly developing adaptive responses. From the previous discussion and other chapters in this volume, it is clear that modern neuroimaging techniques are providing insights into the potential mechanisms underlying functional recovery. These clinical studies complement the fundamental investigations being carried out in the laboratory.

As brain recovery mechanisms are better elucidated, neuroimaging is likely to prove critical in defining which patients might benefit from a specific pharmacologic intervention. Neuroimaging can certainly provide helpful information concerning lesion location. It is currently not possible to identify patients with diaschisis based on clinical criteria. If the resolution of diaschisis proves an important mechanism underlying motor recovery after focal injury to the cortex, then neuroimaging (either positron emission tomography or functional MRI) may provide the sole method of identifying the subgroup of patients likely to benefit from treatments aimed at hastening its reversal. If the activation of latent neural pathways proves important, then functional neuroimaging may help determine which patients may respond to a specific pharmacologic intervention, or which of several interventions may be the most effective.

▉▉▉▉ *Summary*

It is clear that certain drugs influence behavioral recovery in laboratory animals with focal brain injury. These drug effects can be either beneficial or harmful to the recovery process. Importantly, similar drug effects may occur in humans. Therapeutically, drug treatment aimed at hastening recovery will need to be tailored to the individual patient. Subpopulations that might benefit from a specific drug must be identified and issues related to the timing of the intervention and dosing schedules must be clarified through controlled trials. Neuroimaging may help in developing an understanding of the mechanisms of these drug effects on recovery and ultimately help to determine which patients are the most likely to benefit.

References

1. Lincoln NB, Blackburn M, Ellis S, et al. An investigation of factors affecting progress of patients on a stroke unit. *J Neurol Neurosurg Psychiatry* 1989;52:493–96.
2. Feeney DM, Gonzalez A, Law WA. Amphetamine haloperidol and experience interact to affect the rate of recovery after motor cortex injury. *Science* 1982;217:855–57.
3. Hovda DA, Feeney DM. Amphetamine with experience promotes recovery of locomotor function after unilateral frontal cortex injury in the cat. *Brain* 1984;298:358–61.
4. Meyer PM, Horel JA, Meyer DR. Effects of d-amphetamine upon placing responses in neodecorticate cats. *J Comp Physiol Psych* 1963;56:402–404.
5. Sutton RL, Hovda DA, Feeney DM. Amphetamine accelerates recovery of locomotor function following bilateral frontal cortex ablation in cats. *Behav Neurol* 1989;103:837–41.
6. Feeney DM, Hovda DA. Reinstatement of binocular depth perception by amphetamine and visual experience after visual cortex ablation. *Brain Res* 1985;342:352–56.
7. Hovda DA, Sutton RL, Feeney DM. Amphetamine-induced recovery of visual cliff performance after bilateral visual cortex ablation in cats: measurement of depth perception thresholds. *Behav Neurosci* 1989;103:574–84.
8. Goldstein LB. Pharmacology of recovery after stroke. *Stroke* 1990;21 (Suppl III):III-139–III-142.
9. Dunbar GL, Smith GA, Look SK, Whalen RJ. d-amphetamine attenuates learning and motor deficits following cortical injury in rats. *Soc Neurosci Abstr* 1989;15:132.
10. Feeney DM, Sutton RL. Catecholamines and recovery of function after brain damage. In: Stein DG, Sabel BA (eds.). *Pharmacological approaches to the treatment of brain and spinal cord injury.* New York: Plenum Publishing Corp., 1988:121–42.
11. Dietrich WD, Alonso O. Busto R, Ginsberg MD. Influence of amphetamine treatment on somatosensory function of the normal and infarcted rat brain. *Stroke* 1990;21 (Suppl III):III-147–III-150.
12. Colbourne F. Corbett D. Effects of d-amphetamine on the recovery of function following cerebral ischemic injury. *Pharmacol Biochem Behav* 1992;42:705–10.
13. Goldstein LB, Davis JN. Post-lesion practice and amphetamine-facilitated recovery of beam-walking in the rat. *Restorative Neurol Neurosci* 1990;1:311–14.
14. Fuxe K, Ungerstedt U. Histochemical, biochemical and functional studies on central monoamine neurons after acute and chronic amphetamine administration. In: Costa E, Garattini S (eds.). *Amphetamines and related compounds.* New York: Raven Press, 1970:257–88.

15. Hovda DA, Bailey B, Montoya S, Salo AA, Feeney DM. Phentermine accelerates recovery of function after motor cortex injury in rats and cats. *Fed Am Soc Exp Biol* 1983;42:1157.

16. Chen MJ, Sutton RL, Feeney DM. Recovery of function after brain injury in rat and cat: beneficial effects of phenylpropanolamine. *Soc Neurosci Abstr* 1986;12:881.

17. Feeney Dm, Sutton RL. Pharmacotherapy for recovery of function after brain injury. *CRC Crit Rev Neurobiol* 1987;3:135–97.

18. Kline AE, Flores TP, Tso-Olivas DY, Chen MJ, Feeney DM. Effects of methylphenidate on recovery from ablation-induced hemiplegia. *Soc Neurosci Abstr* 1988;14:1152.

19. Goldstein LB. Amphetamine-facilitated functional recovery after stroke. In: Ginsberg MD, Dietrich WD (eds.). *Cerebrovascular diseases*. Sixteenth Research (Princeton) Conference. New York: Raven Press, 1989:303–308.

20. Goldstein LB, Poe HV, Davis JN. An animal model of recovery of function after stroke: facilitation of recovery by an α2-adrenergic receptor antagonist. *Ann Neurol* 1989;26:157.

21. Weaver MS, Farmer LJ, Feeney DM. Norepinephrine receptor agonists and antagonists influence rate and maintenance of recovery of function after sensorimotor cortex contusion in the rat. *Soc Neurosci Abstr* 1987;13:477.

22. Sutton RL, Feeney DM. α-noradrenergic agonists and antagonists affect recovery and maintenance of beam-walking ability after sensorimotor cortex ablation in the rat. *Restorative Neurol Neurosci* 1992;4:1-11.

23. Goldstein LB, Davis JN. Clonidine impairs recovery of beam-walking in rats. *Brain Res* 1990;508:305–309.

24. Stephens J, Goldberg G, Demopoulos JT. Clonidine reinstates deficits following recovery from sensorimotor cortex lesions in rats. *Arch Phys Med Rehabil* 1986;67:666–67.

25. Feeney DM, Westerberg VS. Norepinephrine and brain damage: alpha noradrenergic pharmacology alters functional recovery after cortical trauma. *Can J Psychol* 1990;44:233–52.

26. Hovda DA, Feeney DM, Salo AA, Boyeson MG. Phenoxybenzamine but not haloperidol reinstates all motor and sensory deficits in cats fully recovered from sensorimotor cortex ablations. *Soc Neurosci Abstr* 1983;9:1002.

27. Van Hasselt P. Effect of butyrophenomes on motor function in rats after recovery from brain damage. *Neuropharmacology* 1973;12:2445–47.

28. Hovda DA, Feeney DM. Haloperidol blocks amphetamine induced recovery of binocular depth perception after bilateral visual cortex ablation in the cat. *Proc West Pharmacol Soc* 1985;28:209–11.

29. Davis JN, Arnett CD, Hoyler E, Stalvey LP, Daly JW, Skolnick P. Brain alpha-adrenergic receptors: comparison of [3H]WB4101 binding with norepinephrine-simulated cyclic AMP accumulation in rat cerebral cortex. *Brain Res* 1978;159:125–35.

30. Peroutka SJ. U'Pritchard DC, Greenberg DA, Snyder SH. Neuroleptic drug interactions with norepinephrine alpha receptor binding sites in rat brain. *Neuropharmacology* 1977;16:549–56.

31. Cohen BM, Lipinski JF. In vivo potencies of antipsychotic drugs in blocking alpha 1 noradrenergic and dopamine D2 receptors: implications for drug mechanisms of action. *Life Sciences* 1986;39:2571–80.

32. Boyeson MG, Feeney DM. Intraventricular norepinephrine facilitates motor recovery following sensorimotor cortex injury. *Pharmacol Biochem Behav* 1990;35:497–501.

33. Boyeson MG, Harmon RI. Effects of trazodone and desipramine on motor recovery in brain-injured rats. *Am J Phys Med Rehabil* 1993;72:286–93.

34. Nyback HV, Walters JR, Aghajanian GK, Roth RH. Tricyclic antidepressants: effects on the firing rate of brain noradrenergic neurons. *Eur J Pharmacol* 1975;32:303–12.

35. Svensson TH, Usdin T. Feedback inhibition of brain noradrenaline neurons by tricyclic antidepressants: α-receptor mediation. *Science* 1978;202:1089–91.

36. Roffler-Tarlov S, Schildkraut JJ, Draskoczy PR. Effects of acute and chronic administration of desmethylimipramine on the content of norepinephrine and other monamines in the rat brain. *Biochem Pharmacol* 1973;22:2923–26.

37. Brailowsky S, Knight RT, Blood H. γ-aminobutyric acid-induced potentiation of cortical hemiplegia. *Brain Res* 1986;362:322–30.

38. Schallert T, Hernandez TD, Barth TM. Recovery of function after brain damage: severe and chronic disruption by diazepam. *Brain Res* 1986;379:104–11.

39. Hernandez TD, Kiefel J, Barth TM, Grant ML, Schallert T. Disruption and facilitation of recovery of behavioral function: implication of the gamma-aminobutyric acid/benzodiazepine receptor complex. In: Ginsberg MD, Dietrich WD (eds.). *Cerebrovascular diseases*. Sixteenth Research (Princeton) Conference. New York: Raven Press, 1989:327–34.

40. Moratalla R, Barth TM, Bowery NG. Benzodiazepine receptor autoradiography in corpus striatum of rat after frontal cortex lesion and chronic diazepam treatment. *Neuropharmacology* 1989;28:893–900.

41. Hernandez TD, Schallert T. Long-term impairment of behavioral recovery from cortical damage can be produced by short-term GABA-agonist infusion into adjacent cortex. *Restorative Neurol Neurosci* 1990;1:323–30.

42. Hernandez TD, Jones GH, Schallert T. Co-administration of Ro 15-1788 prevents diazepam-induced retardation of recovery of function. *Brain Res* 1989;487:89–95.

43. Schallert T, Jones TA, Weaver MS, Shapiro LE, Crippens D, Fulton R. Pharmacologic and anatomic considerations in recovery of function. *Phys Med Rehab* 1992;6:375–95.

44. Brailowsky S, Knight RT, Efron R. Phenytoin increases the severity of cortical hemiplegia in rats. *Brain Res* 1986;376:71–77.

45. Chweh AY, Swinyard EA, Wolf HH. Involvement of a GABAergic mechanism in the pharmacologic action of phenytoin. *Pharmacol Biochem Behav* 1986;24:1301–1304.

46. Hernandez TD, Holling LC. Disruption of behavioral recovery by the anti-convulsant phenobarbital. *Brain Res* 1994;635:300–306.

47. Watson CW, Kennard MA. The effect of anticonvulsant drugs on recovery of function following cerebral cortical lesions. *J Neurophysiol* 1945;8:221–31.

48. Fulton RL, Schallert T. Effects of carbamazepine on recovery after cortical damage. *Soc Neurosci Abstr* 1989;15:782.

49. Goldstein LB, Coviello A. Post-lesion administration of the NMDA receptor antagonist MK-801 does not impair motor recovery after unilateral sensorimotor cortex injury in the rat. *Brain Res* 1992;580:129–36.

50. Barth TM, Grant ML, Schallert T. Effects of MK-801 on recovery from sensorimotor cortex lesions. *Stroke* 1990;21 (Suppl III):III-153–III-157.

51. Ward AA Jr, Kennard MA. Effect of cholinergic drugs on recovery of function following lesions of the central nervous system in monkeys. *Yale J Biol & Med* 1942;15:189–228.

52. De Ryck M, Duytschaever H, Janssen PAJ. Ionic channels, cholinergic mechanisms, and recovery of sensorimotor function after neocortical infarcts in rats. *Stroke* 1990;21 (Suppl III):III-158–III-163.

53. Hayes RL, Lyeth BG, Dixon CE, Stonnington HH, Becker DP. Cholinergic antagonist reduces neurologic deficits following cerebral concussion in the rat. *J Cereb Blood Flow Metab* 1985;5 (Suppl1):S395–S396.

54. Saponjic RM, Barbay S. Hoane MR, Irish SL, Barth TM. Scopolamine facilitates recovery of forelimb placing behavior following unilateral cortical lesions in the rat. *Soc Neurosci Abstr* 1993;19:1012.

55. Held JM, Gordon J, Gentile AM. Environmental influences on locomotor recovery following cortical lesions in rats. *Behav Neurosci* 1985;99:678–90.

56. Stephens J. Effects of assistance, practice, and learning on recovery from sensorimotor cortex lesions in rats. *Soc Neurosci Abstr* 1986;12:1285.

57. Stephens J. Rat model for studying recovery from brain injury: training and assistance facilitate recovery. *Phys Ther* 1986;66:781–80.

58. Goldstein LB, Davis JN. Post-lesion practice and amphetamine-facilitated recovery of beam-walking in the rat. *Restorative Neurol Neurosci* 1990;1:311-14.

59. Bliss TVP, Dolphin AC. What is the mechanism of long-term potentiation in the hippocampus? *TINS* 1982;5:289–90.

60. Bliss TVP, Lomo T. Long-lasting potentiation of synaptic transmission in the dentate area of the anaesthetized rabbit following stimulation of the perforant path. *J Physiol* 1973; 232:331–56.

61. Bliss TVP, Gardner-Medwin AR. Long-lasting potentiation of synaptic transmission in the dentate area of the unanaesthetized rabbit following stimulation of the perforant path. *J Physiol* 1973;232:357–74.

62. Corbett D. Long term potentiation of lateral hypothalamic self-stimulation following parabrachial lesions in the rat. *Brain Res Bull* 1980;5:637–42.

63. Artola A, Singer W. NMDA receptors and developmental plasticity in visual neocortex. In: Collingridge GL, Watkins JC (eds.). *The NMDA receptor.* Oxford: Oxford University Press, 1989:153–66.

64. Aroniadou VA, Teyler TJ. The role of NMDA receptors in long-term potentiation (LTP) and depression (LTD) in rat visual cortex. *Brain Res* 1991;562:136–43.

65. Keller A, Iriki A, Asanuma H. Identification of neurons producing long-term potentiation in the cat motor cortex: intracellular recordings and labeling. *J Comp Neurol* 1990;300:47–60.

66. Wall PD. Mechanisms of plasticity of connection following damage in adult mammalian nervous systems. In: Bach-y-Rita P (ed.). *Recovery of function: theoretical considerations for brain injury rehabilitation.* Baltimore: University Park Press, 1978;91–105.

67. Chollet F, DiPiero V, Wise RJS, Brooks DJ, Dolan RJ, Frackowiak RSJ. The functional anatomy of motor recovery after stroke in humans: a study with positron emission tomography. *Ann Neurol* 1991;29:63–71.

68. Weiller C, Chollet F, Friston KJ, Wise RJS, Frackowiak RSJ. Functional reorganization of the brain in recovery from striatocapsular infarction in man. *Ann Neurol* 1992;31:463–72.

69. Weiller C, Ramsay SC, Wise RJS, Friston KJ, Frackowiak RSJ. Individual patterns of functional reorganization in the human cerebral cortex after capsular infarction. *Ann Neurol* 1993;33:181–89.

70. von Monakow C. *Die lokalisation im grosshirn und der abbau der funktion durch kortikale herde.* Wiesbaden: J.F. Bergmann, 1914.

71. Jaspers RMA, Van Der Sprenkel JWB, Tulleken CAF, Cools AR. Local as well as remote functional and metabolic changes after focal ischemia in cats. *Brain Res Bull* 1990; 24:23–32.

72. Theodore DR, Meier-Ruge W, Abraham J. Microvascular morphometry in primate diaschisis. *Microvas Res* 1992;43:147–55.

73. Castella Y, Dietrich WD, Watson BD, Busto R. Acute thrombotic infarction suppresses metabolic activation of ipsilateral somatosensory cortex: evidence for functional diaschisis. *J Cereb Blood Flow Metab* 1989;9:329–41.

74. Feeney DM, Sutton RL, Boyeson MG, Hovda DA, Dail WG. The locus-coeruleus and cerebral metabolism: recovery of function after cortical injury. *Physiol Psych* 1985;13:197–203.

75. Feeney DM. Pharmacologic modulation of recovery after brain injury: a reconsideration of diasachisis. *J Neuro Rehab* 1991;5:113–28.

76. Lenzi GL, Frackowiak RSJ, Jones T. Cerebral oxygen metabolism and blood flow in human cerebral infarction. *J Cereb Blood Flow Metab* 1982;2:321.

77. Martin WRW, Raichle ME. Cerebellar blood flow and metabolism in cerebral hemisphere infarction. *Ann Neurol* 1983;14:168–76.

78. Fiorelli M, Blin J, Bakchine S, Laplane D, Baron JC. PET studies of cortical diaschisis in patients with motor hemi-neglect. *J Neurol Sci* 1991;104:135–42.

79. Tanaka M, Kondo S, Hirai S, Isgiguro K, Ishihara T, Morimatsu M. Crossed cerebellar diaschisis accompanied by hemiataxia: a PET study. *J Neurol Neurosurg Psychiatry* 1992; 55:121–25.

80. Boetz MI, Leveille J, Lambert R, Boetz T. Single photon emission tomography (SPECT) in cerebellar disease: cerebello-cerebral diaschisis. *Eur Neurol* 1991;31:405–12.

81. Pappata S, Mazoyer B, Dinh T, Cambon H, Levasseur M, Baron JC. Effects of capsular or thalamic stroke on metabolism in the cortex and cerebellum: a positron emission tomography study. *Stroke* 1991;21:519–24.

82. Steward O. Reorganization of neuronal connections following CNA trauma: principles and experimental paradigms. *J Neurotrauma* 1989;6:99–152.

83. Lipton SA, Kater SB. Neurotransmitter regulation of neuronal outgrowth, plasticity and survival. *TINS* 1989;12:265–70.

84. Clark ANG, Mankikar GD. d-amphetamine in elderly patients refractory to rehabilitation procedures. *J Am Geriatr Soc* 1979;27:174–77.

85. Crisotomo EA, Duncan PW, Propst MA, Dawson DB, Davis JN. Evidence that amphetamine with physical therapy promotes recovery of motor function in stroke patients. *Ann Neurol* 1988;23:94–97.

86. Fugl-Meyer AR, Jaasko L, Leyman I, Olsson S, Steglind S. The post-stroke hemiplegic patient. I. A method for evaluation of physical performance. *Scand J Rehab Med* 1975; 7:13–31.

87. Borucki SJ, Langberg J, Reding M. The effect of dextroamphetamine on motor recovery after stroke. *Neurology* 1992;42 (Suppl 3):329.

88. Walker-Batson D, Smith P, Curtis S, et al. Amphetamine paired with physical therapy accelerates motor recovery following stroke: further evidence. *Stroke* 1995;26:2254-59.

89. Albert ML, Bachman DL, Morgan A, Helm-Estabrooks N. Pharmacotherapy for aphasia. *Neurology* 1988;38:877–79.

90. Bachman DL, Morgan A. The role of pharmacotherapy in the treatment of aphasia. *Aphasiology* 1988;3–4:225–28.

91. Sabe L, Leiguarda R. Starkstein SE. An open-label trial of bromocriptine in nonfluent aphasia. *Neurology* 1992;42:1637–38.

92. Homan R, Panksepp J, Mcsweeny J, et al. d-amphetamine effects on language and motor behaviors in a chronic stroke patient. *Soc Neurosci Abstr* 1990;16:439.

93. Walker-Batson D, Unwin H, Curtis S, et al. Use of amphetamine in the treatment of aphasia. *Restorative Neurol Neurosci* 1992;4:47–50.

94. Morris PLP, Raphael B, Robinson RG. Clinical depression is associated with impaired recovery from stroke. *Med J Aust* 1992;157:239–42.

95. Reding MJ, Orto LA, Winter SW, Fortuna IM, Di Ponte P, McDowell FH. Antidepressant therapy after stroke. A double-blind trial. *Arch Neurol* 1986;43:763–65.

96. Meyer JS, Miyakawa Y, Welch KMA, et al. Influence of adrenergic receptor blockade on circulatory and metabolic effects of disordered neurotransmitter function in stroke patients. *Stroke* 1976;7:158–67.

97. Porch BE, Feeney DM. Effects of antihypertensive drugs on recovery from aphasia. *Clin Aphasiology* 1986;16:309–14.

98. Goldstein LB, Davis JN. Physician prescribing patterns after ischemic stroke. *Neurology* 1988;38:1806–1809.

99. Porch B, Wyckes J, Feeney DM. Haloperidol, thiazides, and some antihypertensives slow recovery from aphasia. *Soc Neurosci Abstr* 1985;11:52.

100. Goldstein LB, Matchar DB, Morgenlander JC, Davis JN. The influence of drugs on the recovery of sensorimotor function after stroke. *J Neuro Rehab* 1990;4:137–44.

101. Goldstein LB, SASS Study Investigators. Common drugs may influence motor recovery after stroke. *Neurology* 1995;45:865-71.

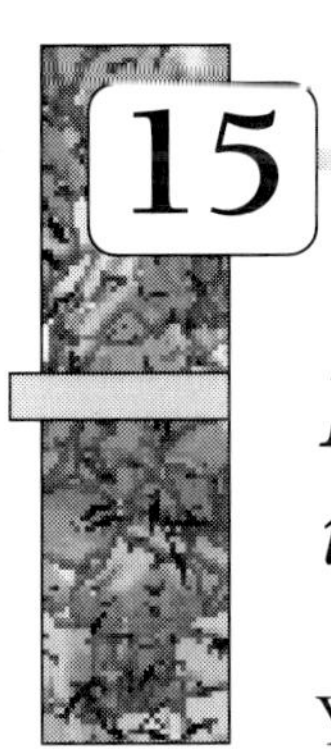

15

Diffusion Mapping in Brain Ischemia

Yasuhiro Hasegawa, M.D., Ph.D.

Introduction

Pulsed field gradient nuclear magnetic resonance is emerging as a powerful tool for experimental and clinical studies of brain ischemia (1,2). With the imposition of pulsed magnetic field gradients onto spin echo magnetic resonance imaging (MRI), molecular displacements, such as diffusion of water due to Brownian motion, can be noninvasively measured. In biological tissue, microscopic structures, such as cell membranes and cellular organelles, impede diffusion, resulting in an apparent diffusion coefficient (ADC) that is less than that of free fluid (3,4). The technique of generating image contrast based on differences of restricted diffusion coefficients of water protons in tissue is known as diffusion-weighted MRI (DWI). Signal intensity measured by the typical Stejskal and Tanner pulse sequence is expressed as the following equation (5):

$$SI = SI_0 exp(-k^2 t D_{app}).$$

Where SI is the signal intensity, SI_0 is the signal without any attenuation, D_{app} is the ADC, k is a variable that is defined by the time integral of the diffusion-sensitizing gradient pulses, and t is a function of the duration of applied gradient and the time between applied pulses. The $k^2 t$ term is customarily referred to as the b-value (3). When combined with an ultrafast imaging technique, such as echo-planar imaging, these techniques can be expanded to allow the quantitation of ADC in a spatially localized fashion, hence "ADC mapping" (6). Briefly, more than two DWIs are obtained with different b-values. ADC mapping can be performed by calculating the slope of the regression line between the $ln(SI/SI_0)$ and b-value on a pixel-by-pixel basis. Cerebral ischemia has been most extensively studied by DWI. It is now well established that the ADC of brain water significantly decreases within a few minutes after the onset of brain ischemia (7–13). The exact mechanism of this reduction in ADC remains unexplained; however, it has been attributed to cytotoxic edema and membrane permeability changes caused by brain energy failure (11,14,15). Evaluation of ischemic damage using DWI during the potentially reversible phase of ischemia may help to develop new strategies for the treatment of stroke patients. An important question to address is whether a certain pathophysiological status of brain tissue can be determined by the information derived from these noninvasive methods.

Evaluation of Ischemic Penumbra by ADC Mapping

The original concept of the ischemic penumbra evolved from the existence of two different thresholds for cessation of electrical activity and the maintenance of transmembrane ionic gradients (16–18). However, some have used this term in a broader sense to denote the potentially reversible perifocal region that may be recruited into the infarction process unless cerebral blood flow (CBF) is restored or other measures are taken that prevent the process of cell death (19,20). The latter concept is more practical and useful in the clinical setting. It has been reported that the reversal of the early hyperintensity by CBF restoration occurs in temporary focal ischemia models (8,10,21). These observations suggested that the hyperintensity seen on early DWI in part represents reversible ischemic tissue injury, i.e., ischemic penumbra. If the varying degree of ADC changes would represent the severity of the ischemic brain tissue damage, diffusion MRI technique could be used to evaluate the ischemic penumbra.

Reduction of the Ischemic Lesion Area with Abnormal ADC by CBF Restoration

We investigated the reversibility of the area with initially reduced ADC values by acquiring ADC maps before and after a transient middle cerebral artery (MCA) occlusion in rats (22). Forty-five minutes of transient MCA occlusion was produced by introducing a nylon suture through the common carotid artery and advancing intracranially to block the origin of the MCA (23,24). CBF was restored by retracting the nylon filament. Figure 15-1A shows the ADC map of a rat brain slice at the optic chiasm level forty minutes after the MCA occlusion. After the CBF restoration, recovery of initially decreased ADC values was observed in the periphery of the lesion and the lesion size was decreased (Figure 15-1B). In contrast, a further decline of ADC values was observed in the core of the lesion. The subtraction of these two images clearly demonstrates the topographical changes (Figure 15-1C). The size and shape of the infarct area determined by TTC staining twenty-four hours after the ischemia coincides well with the region visualized in the ADC map two hours after the reperfusion (Figure 15-1D). ROI analysis was performed on the serial ADC images and the TTC slice image using the image processing software, To negate the regional variability mainly due to anisotropy, regional changes of ADC values were evaluated by ΔADC, defined as the difference between ADC value in an ischemic region and that in a contralateral homologous region. Figure 15-2 is a scatter plot of ΔADC values two hours after the reperfusion against pre-reperfusion values. ΔADC values in 53 ROIs, of which areas were totally infarcted or totally non-infarcted on TTC slice image, were plotted. In this study, the existence of threshold is of special importance, i.e., recovery of initially reduced ADC values occurred only in ischemic regions where ΔADC values did not decrease by more than $-0.25 \times 10^{-5} \text{cm}^2/\text{sec}$. ADC values progressively decreased in regions with initially severely decreased pre-reperfusion ADC values

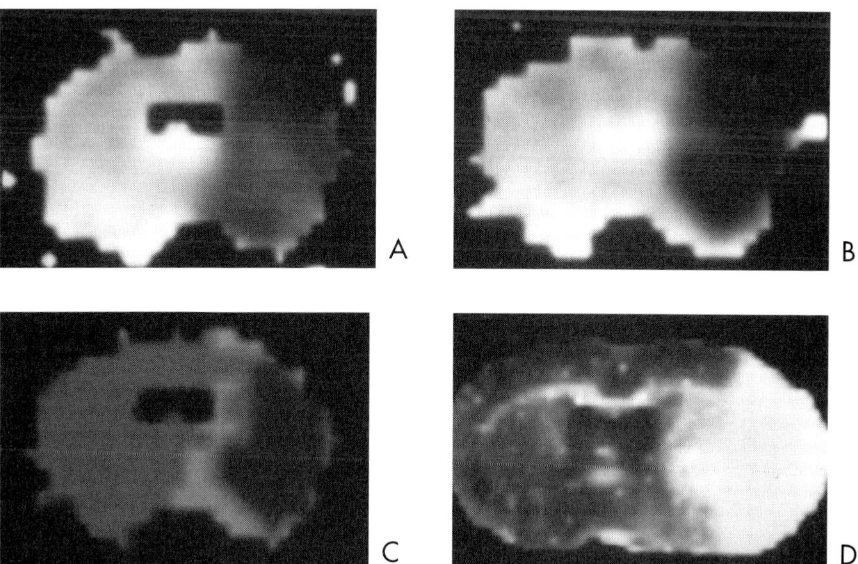

Figure 15-1. Cerebral maps of the apparent diffusion coefficient (ADC) and TTC staining from a rat with forty-five minutes transient middle cerebral artery occlusion. (A) An ADC map obtained forty minutes after occlusion. A gray scale shows the absolute ADC value ($\times 10^{-5}$cm²/sec). (B) An ADC map obtained at 120 minutes post-reperfusion. The gray scale is the same as A. (C) Subtraction image (B–A) using two threshold values, $\pm 0.05 \times 10^{-5}$cm²/sec, based on a variation of the differential values of ADC is the contralateral non-ischemic hemisphere. (D) TTC staining (data from *Neurology* 1994;44:1484).

after reperfusion and postmortem examination always demonstrated infarction in such regions. Thus, ADC measurements can provide information to discriminate between irreversible and potentially reversible ischemic regions before reperfusion is performed.

Three-Dimensional Evolution of Ischemic Lesion

To determine the evolution of ischemic lesion by serial ADC mapping may be another way of approach to explore the possibility that the heterogeneous range of ADC values predicts potential reversibility. Figure 15-3 shows serial multi-slice ADC maps of a rat brain with permanent suture MCA occlusion. The multi-slice ADC mapping was performed by obtaining sixteen sets of DWI under different b-values in each slice. The total acquisition time of images required to calculate the eight-slice ADC maps was approximately one minute. The core of the ischemic lesion showed very low ADC values below 0.40×10^{-5}cm²/sec. During the time of observation, the area with moderately reduced ADC values, which surrounded the ischemic core, evolved into lower ADC values. The ischemic lesion was initially observed in the lateral part of the caudoputamen and the lower part of the frontoparietal cortex, with delayed development

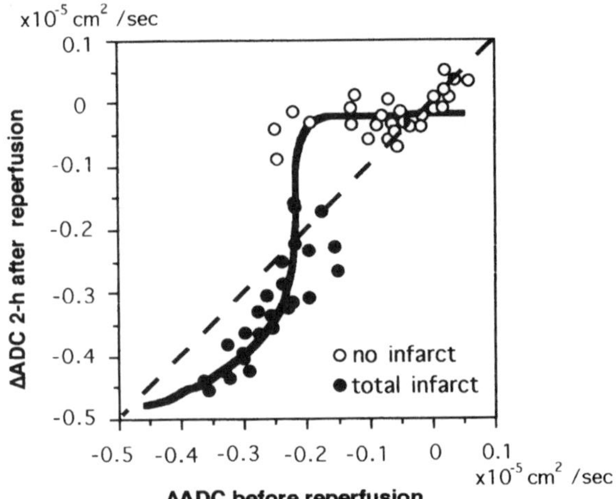

Figure 15-2. The relationship between ΔADC values before (at forty minutes post-occlusion) and 120 minutes after reperfusion of the middle cerebral artery territory. The pathological outcome in each region of interest is indicated by the following symbols: open circle: no infarct; solid circle: totally infarcted. Dotted line: line of identity. Solid line represents the relationship between pre- and post-reperfusion ΔADC values (modified data from *Neurology* 1994;44:1484).

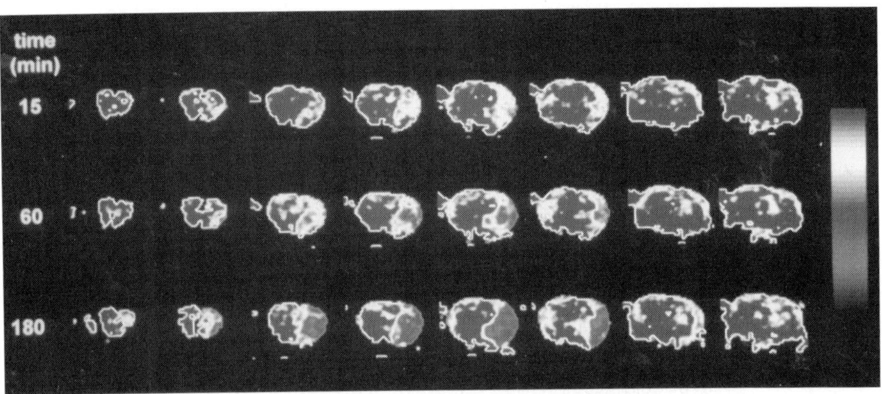

Figure 15-3. Three-dimensional evolution of ischemic damage.

in the frontal and occipital parts of the brain. The ischemic lesion volume with abnormally low ADC values ($< 0.55 \times 10^{-5}$cm²/sec) increases over time and reaches almost plateau at about two to three hours after the MCA occlusion. The ischemic lesion volume three hours after the MCA occlusion was well correlated with postmortem infarct volume determined by TTC staining (25). The areas showing normal ADC values in the frontal and occipital part of the brain subsequently evolved to the ischemic lesion areas, implying that the ischemic penumbra may be larger than the region where the initially reduced ADC recovered after the reperfusion.

Cortical Spreading Depression

Cortical spreading depression of Leão (SD) (26–28) represents a spontaneously reversible failure of brain ion homeostasis accompanied by a depolarization of neurons and glial cells, which spreads across the cortical surface from its initiation site as a wave with a speed of 2–5 mm/min (29–31). SD is elicitable by a number of chemical, mechanical, and electrical stimuli in normal brain and is spontaneously elicited in several brain diseases. It is well known that SD or SD-like spontaneous depolarization occurs in cortical regions surrounding an acute ischemic lesion (32–36). The number of DC deflections correlates with ultimate infarct volume and suppression of DC deflection by a glutamate antagonist or brain temperature modulation decreases infarct volume (32,33,37). Therefore, SD may contribute to progression of the ischemic process including ischemic penumbra. During SD, redistribution of ions and water occurs in the intra- and extracellular space, resulting in the shrinkage of the extracellular space by 50% (38,39). The shift of tissue water from the extra- to intracellular space during SD should restrict the translational movement of water molecules and cause a local decline in the ADC of water. As shown in Figures 15-4 and 15-5, diffusion MRI can noninvasively depict a ripple-like movement of SD in normal an

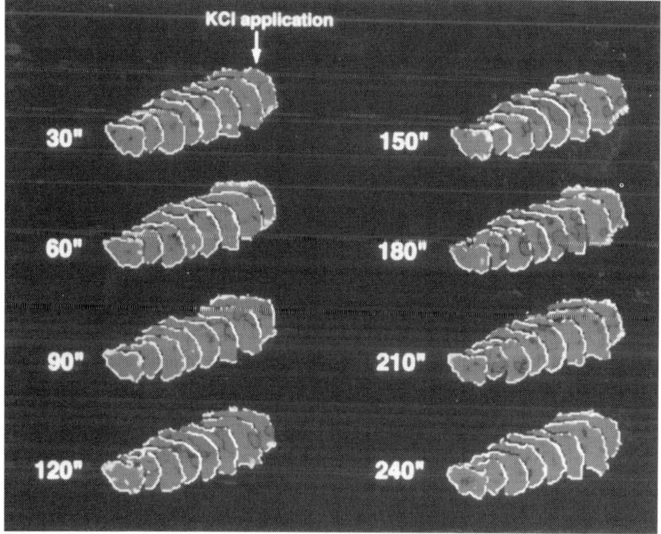

Figure 15-4 Spreading depression in normal brain. To demonstrate the propagation of regions with decreased apparent diffusion coefficients, the eight contiguous maps (1.5 mm thick) were stacked and the areas with abnormally decreased ADC pixel values ($< 0.55 \times 10^{-5}$ cm²/sec) were displayed as a blue area. Topical application of potassium chloride (*arrow*) elicits a ripple-like movement of waves of decreased ADC.

ischemic rat brain as a wave of decreased ADC (40,41). Especially in the ischemic brain, we can evaluate the effect of a single passage of wave of decreased ADC on the ischemic lesion size (Figure 15-5). Although well-documented under experimental conditions, the role of SD in human stroke is still a matter of speculation because the human cortex is not as susceptible to SD as the rodent and cats. If the occurrence of SD is a phenomenon specific to experimental stroke, then the observations obtained from animal models highly susceptible to SD should be cautiously interpreted. If SD also occurs in stroke patients, its relevance to clinical focal ischemia can be studied. Multi-slice echo-planar DWI with ultrafast imaging technique is already available to human stroke. These new MRI technologies should reveal the contribution of SD in human stroke in the near future.

■■■■ Conclusion

In spite of a large number of experimental studies, the pathophysiology of brain ischemia has not been completely understood and no specific therapy has been established yet. Recent experimental studies have shed some light on therapeutic strategies, such as reperfusion by tissue plasminogen activator, inhibition of excitatory amino acids, inhibition of SD, and brain temperature modulation, etc. Clinical application of diffusion MRI techniques may help to develop such a new therapy of acute ischemic

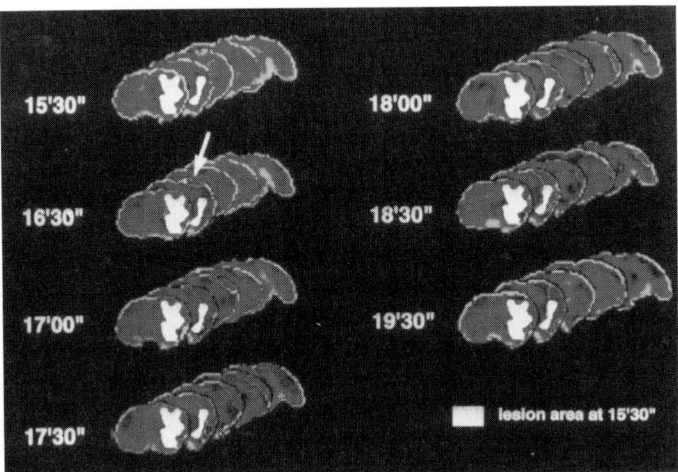

Figure 15-5. Spreading depression in ischemic brain. Five contiguous ADC maps were stacked. Initially, ischemic lesions were observed in the caudate-putamen and adjacent cortex at 15.5 minutes post-occlusion. At l6.5 minutes post-occlusion, a small region with decreased ADC values appeared in the patrietal cortex (*arrow*), distinct from the likely evolving ischemic lesion. This separate region with decreased ADC values then spread over the cortex, propagating posteriorly over the next two minutes and then disappeared by the 19.5 minute time point.

stroke by determining the ischemic lesion size before and after the intervention (42,43). The MRI technology also may help to visualize certain pathological conditions, such as SD, of which contribution to human brain diseases has been evaluated only in the experimental condition.

Acknowledgments: I gratefully acknowledge Dr. Marc Fisher for his critical review of the manuscript.

References

1. Fisher M, Minematsu K. Novel magnetic resonance studies for acute stroke: the dawn of a new era. *Cerebrovasc Dis* 1992;2:253–55.
2. Fisher M, Sotak CH, Minematsu K, Li L. New magnetic resonance techniques for evaluating cerebrovascular disease. *Ann Neurol* 1992;32:115–21.
3. LeBihan D, Breton E, Lallemand D, Grenier P, Cabanis E, Leval-Jeantet M. MR imaging of intravoxel incoherent motions: application to diffusion and perfusion in neurologic disorders. *Radiology* 1986;161:401–407.
4. LeBihan D. Molecular diffusion nuclear magnetic resonance imaging. *Magn Reson* 1991;Q7:1–30.
5. Stejskal EO, Tanner JE. Spin diffusion measurements: spin echoes in the presence of a time-dependent field gradient. *J Chem Phys* 1965;42:288–92.
6. Dardzinski BJ, Sotak CH, Fisher M, Hasegawa Y, Li L, Minematsu K. Apparent diffusion coefficient mapping of experimental focal cerebral ischemia using diffusion-weighted echo-planar imaging. *Magn Reson Med* 1993;30:318–25.
7. Moseley ME, Kucharczyk J, Kurhanewicz J, Norman D. Diffusion-weighted MR imaging of acute stroke: correlation with T2-weighted and magnetic susceptibility-enhanced MR imaging in cats. *Am J Neurorad* 1990;11:423–29.
8. Mintorovitch J, Moseley ME, Chileuitt L, Shimizu H, Cohen Y, Weinstein PR. Comparison of diffusion- and T2-weighted MRI for the early detection of cerebral ischemia and reperfusion in rats. *Magn Reson Med* 1991;18:39–50.
9. Minematsu K, Li L, Fisher M, Sotak CH, Davis MA, Fiandaca MS. Diffusion-weighted magnetic resonance imaging rapid and quantitative detection of focal brain ischemia. *Neurology* 1992;42:235–40.
10. Minematsu K, Li L, Sotak CH, Davis MA, Fisher M. Reversible focal ischemic injury demonstrated by diffusion-weighted magnetic resonance imaging. *Stroke* 1992;23:1304–11.
11. Benveniste H, Hedlund LW, Johnson GA. Mechanism of detection of acute cerebral ischemia in rats by diffusion-weighted magnetic resonance microscopy. *Stroke* 1992;23:746–54.
12. Davis D, Ulatowski J, Eleff S, Izuta M, Mori S, Shungu D, van Zijl DCM. Rapid monitoring of changes in water diffusion coefficients during reversible ischemia in cat and rat brain. *Magn Reson Med* 1994;31:454–60.
13. Warach S, Gaa J, Siewert B, Wielopolski P, Edelman RR. Acute human stroke studied by whole brain echo planar diffusion-weighted magnetic resonance imaging. *Ann Neurol* 1995;37:231–41.
14. Moseley ME, Cohen Y, Mintorovitch J, et al. Early detection of cerebral ischemia in cats: comparison of diffusion- and T2-weighted MRI and spectroscopy. *Magn Reson Med* 1990;14:330–46.

15. Helpern JA, Ordidge RJ, Knight RA. The effect of cell membrane water permeability on the diffusion coefficient of water. *Proceedings of the XI Annual Meeting of the Society of Magnetic Resonance in Medicine* 1992;1:1201.

16. Symon L. The relationship between CBF, evoked potentials and the clinical features in cerebral ischemia. *Acta Neurol Scand* 1980;78(Suppl 78):175–90.

17. Astrup J, Siesjö BK, Symon L. Thresholds in cerebral ischemia—the ischemic penumbra. *Stroke* 1981;12:723–25.

18. Hakim AM. The cerebral ischemic penumbra. *Can J Neurol Sci* 1987;14:557–59.

19. Siesjö BK. Pathophysiology and treatment of focal cerebral ischemia. Part I: Pathophysiology. *J Neurosurg* 1992;77:169–84.

20. Memezawa H, Smith ML, Siesjö BK. Penumbral tissues salvaged by reperfusion following middle cerebral artery occlusion in rats. *Stroke* 1992;23:552–59.

21. Minematsu K, Fisher M, Li L, Sotak CH. Diffusion and perfusion MRI studies to evaluate a non-competitive NMDA antagonist and reperfusion in experimental stroke. *Stroke* 1993;24:2074–81.

22. Hasegawa Y, Fisher M, Latour LL, Dardzinski BJ, Sotak CH. MRI diffusion mapping of reversible and irreversible ischemic injury in focal brain ischemia. *Neurology* 1994;44:1484–90.

23. Koizumi J, Yoshida Y, Nakazawa T, Ooneda G. Experimental studies of ischemic brain edema. 1. A New experimental model of cerebral embolism in rats in which recirculation can be introduced in the ischemic area (in Japanese with English abstract). *Jpn J Stroke* 1986;8:1–8.

24. Zea Longa E, Weinstein PR, Carlson S, Cummins R. Reversible middle cerebral artery occlusion without craniectomy in rats. *Stroke* 1989;20:84–91.

25. Reith W, Hasegawa Y, Latour LL, Dardzinski BJ, Sotak CH, Fisher M. Multislice diffusion mapping for 3-D evolution of cerebral ischemia in a rat stroke model. *Neurology* 1995;45:172–77.

26. Leão AAP. Spreading depression of activity in the cerebral cortex. *J Neurophysiol* 1944;7:359–90.

27. Leão AAP. Further observations on the spreading depression of activity in the cerebral cortex. *J Neurophysiol* 1947;10:409–14.

28. Leão AAP. The slow voltage variation of cortical spreading depression of activity. *Electroencephalogr Clin Neurophysiol* 1951;3:315–21.

29. Marshall WH. Spreading cortical depresssion of Leão. *Physiol Rev* 1959;39:239-79.

30. Hansen AJ, Zeuthen T. Changes in brain extracellular ions during spreading depression. *Acta Physiol Scand* 1981;113:437–45.

31. Somjen GG, Aitken PG, Czàh GL, Herreras O, Jing J, Young JN, Mechanisms of spreading depression: a review of recent findings and a hypothesis. *Can J Physiol Pharmacol* 1992;70:S248–S254.

32. Gill R, Andine P, Hillered L, Persson L, Hagberg H. The efect of MK-801 on cortical spreading depression in the penumbral zone following focal ischemia in the rat. *J Cereb Blood Flow Metab* 1992;12:371–97.

33. Iijima T, Mies G, Hossmann K-A. Repeated negative DC deflections in the rat cortex following middle cerebral artery occlusion are abolished by MK-801: effect on volume of ischemic injury. *J Cereb Blood Flow Metab* 1992;12:717–33.

34. Nedergaard M, Hansen AJ. Characterization of cortical depolarizations evoked in focal cerebral ischemia. *J Cereb Blood Flow Metab* 1993;13:568–74.

35. Bak T, Kohno K, Hossmann KA. Cortical negative DC deflections following middle cere-

bral artery occlusion and KC1-induced spreading depression: effect on blood flow, tissue oxygenation, and electroencephalogram. *J Cereb Blood Flow Metab* 1994;14:12–19.

36. Dietrich WD, Feng Z, Leistra H, Watson BD, Rosenthal M. Photothrombotic infarction triggers multiple episodes of cortical spreading depression in distant brain regions. *J Cereb Blood Flow Metab* 1994;14:20–28.

37. Chen Q, Chopp M, Bodzin G, Chen H. Temperature modulation of cerebral depolarization during focal cerebral ischemia in rats: correlation with ischemic injury. *J Cereb Blood Flow Metab* 1993;13:389–94.

38. van Harreveld A, Khattab FI. Changes in cortical extracellular space during spreading depression investigated with electron microscope. *J Neurophysiol* 1967;30:911–29.

39. Hansen AJ, Olsen CE. Brain extracellular space during spreading depression and ischemia. *Acta Physiol Scand* 1980;108:355–65.

40. Latour LL, Hasegawa Y, Formato JE, Fisher M, Sotak CH. Spreading wave of decreased diffusion coefficient after cortical stimulation in the rat brain. *Magn Reson Med* 1994; 32:189–98.

41. Hasegawa Y, Latour LL, Formato JE, Sotak CH, Fisher M. Spreading waves of a reduced diffusion coefficient of water in normal and ischemic rat brain. *J Cereb Blood Flow Metab* 1995;15:179–87.

42. Minematsu K, Fisher M, Li L, Davis MA, Knapp AG, Cotter RE, McBurney RN, Sotak CH. Effects of a novel NMDA antagonist on experimental stroke rapidly and quantitatively assessed by diffusion-weighted MRI. *Neurology* 1993;43:397–403.

43. Hasegawa Y, Latour LL, Sotak CH, Dardzinski BJ, Fisher M. Temperature dependent change of apparent diffusion coefficient of water in normal and ischemic brain in rats. *J Cereb Blood Flow Metab* 1994;14:383–90.

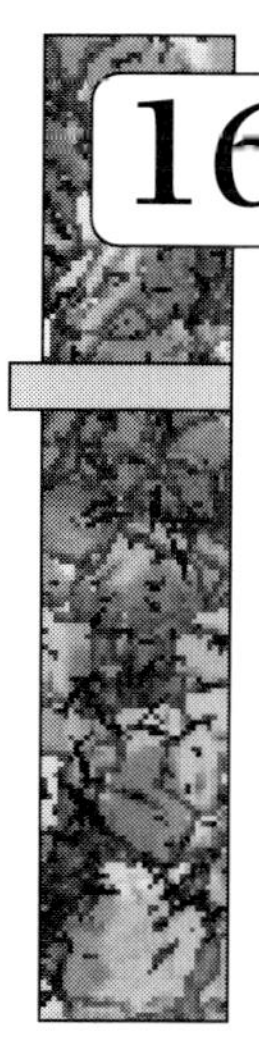

16

Early Spontaneous Reperfusion in Stroke Is a Favorable Prognostic Sign: A SPECT Study

Henrik Stig Jørgensen, M.D., Bjørn Sperling, M.D., Hirofumi Nakayama, M.D., Ph.D., Tom Skyhøj Olsen, M.D., Ph.D., and Niels Alexander Lassen, M.D., Ph.D.

Imaging techniques such as SPECT and PET have shown that the areas affected by an arterial occlusion or a hematoma are usually considerably larger than the structural lesion demonstrated by CT scan. The hemodynamic and metabolic changes occurring outside the actual lesion are mainly explained by diaschisis or an ischemic penumbra (1). The penumbral zone is of particular interest. Whether this zone survives and regains function depends on two factors: collateral circulation and reperfusion due to spontaneous disobliteration of the occluding material (1).

Dalal (1965) (2) showed that half of the stroke patients with occlusion in the carotid territory experienced spontaneous reperfusion within the first five days poststroke. This observation has later been confirmed by several investigators (1). Spontaneous reperfusion is accompanied by markedly increased blood flow in the previously ischemic area to levels sometimes two and three times higher than normal, i.e., luxury perfusion (1,3). It has been debated whether reperfusion with luxury perfusion was a good or bad event. Reperfusion of the penumbral zone might restore neuronal function in the area and reduce the neurologic deficit. On the other hand, hyperperfusion might give rise to blood engorgement and edema and transform the ischemic infarct into a hemorrhagic infarct. This might harm perfusion in the penumbra and worsen clinical outcome (1).

Hyperperfusion due to spontaneous recanalisation has attracted considerable pathophysiological interest. From a clinical point of view, demonstration of the phenomenon has not until recently been considered of significant use in the single patient. It has not been clear if it was of any clinical significance and the demonstration relied on invasive procedures. The introduction of SPECT scanners and their availability for routine clinical purposes have now made it possible to noninvasively monitor brain perfusion and it appears now that spontaneous reperfusion evidenced by focal hyperemia is of significant clinical importance (4).

Patients and Methods

We studied 354 unselected patients with acute ischemic stroke in whom one or more SPECT examinations were performed during hospital stay. ^{99m}Tc-labeled d,1-hexamethylenepropyleneamineoxime=HMPAO with 550 MBq (Ceretec®) injected intravenously was used as a flow tracer (5). Mean age of the patients was 73 years and median time from stroke to admission was ten hours. A CT scan was performed in all patients. Cortical involvement was demonstrated in 146 patients; in 133 patients the infarct was subcortical, while 75 had normal scans. The patients were all assessed clinically on admission, one and two weeks after admission, and at discharge after completion of rehabilitation in a stroke rehabilitation unit using the Scandinavian Stroke Scale (SSS score; 0–58 points).

Results

Spontaneous recanalisation evidenced by focal hyperemia in the infarct area was seen in 77 percent of the patients with cortical infarcts (Figure 16-1). We were not able to demonstrate this phenomenon in patients with subcortical infarcts. The frequency of reperfusion increased rapidly from zero at the time of onset to 30 percent at day 3, and 60 percent at day 7, reaching a maximum on day 14, at which time 77 percent showed reperfusion (Figure 16-2). The hyperperfused state lasted two to three weeks. Hyperperfusion was present at the time of CT scan in twenty patients. A hemorrhage

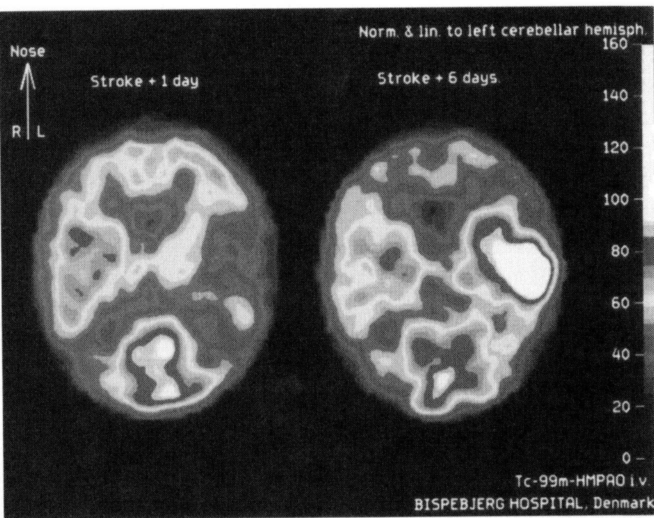

Figure 16-1. Single photon emission computed tomographic examination in a patient with reperfusion. Hyperperfusion followed initial hypoperfusion [from reference (4)].

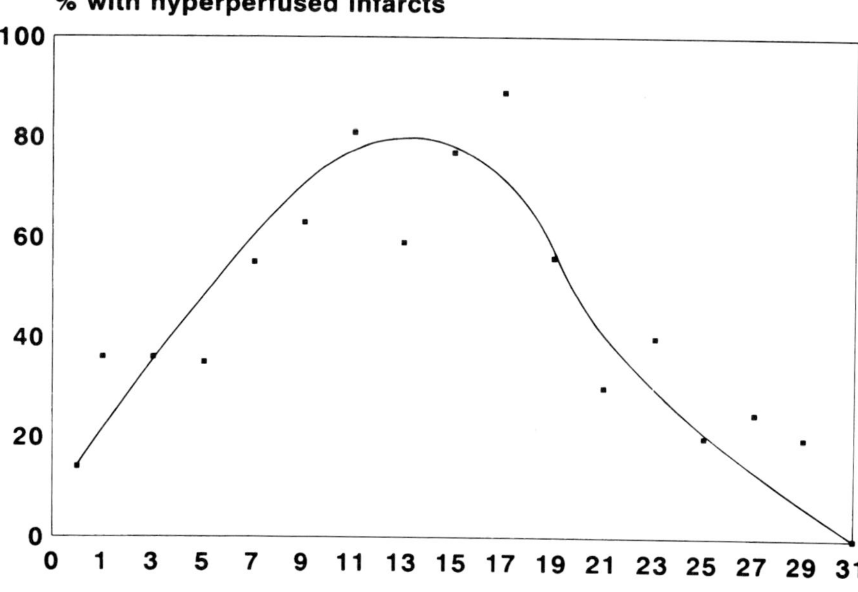

Figure 16-2. Frequency of spontaneously hyperperfused cortical infarcts the first month after stroke onset [from reference (4)].

in the infarct (a hemorrhagic infarct) was present in only four (20 percent) of these twenty patients. The hemorrhages were seen as small, hyperdense spots. No large confluent hematomas, edemas, or mass effect were observed.

We studied clinical outcome in a subgroup of seventeen patients admitted on the first day of stroke in whom recanalisation took place within the first week from stroke onset and nineteen patients in whom the occlusion persisted throughout the first week. These two groups were comparable in age, time from onset to admission, clinical features, and total SSS score on admission. The patients who had spontaneous recanalisation within the first week improved markedly during rehabilitation, whereas patients without reperfusion within the first week showed no clinical improvement (Figure 16-3).

Conclusion

Spontaneous reperfusion per se of the infarcted area cannot account for the marked difference in recovery between the two groups. Most likely the improvement is secondary to reperfusion of the ischemic penumbra leading to normalization of neuronal function in the penumbra, decreasing neurologic deficits. Our findings indicate that

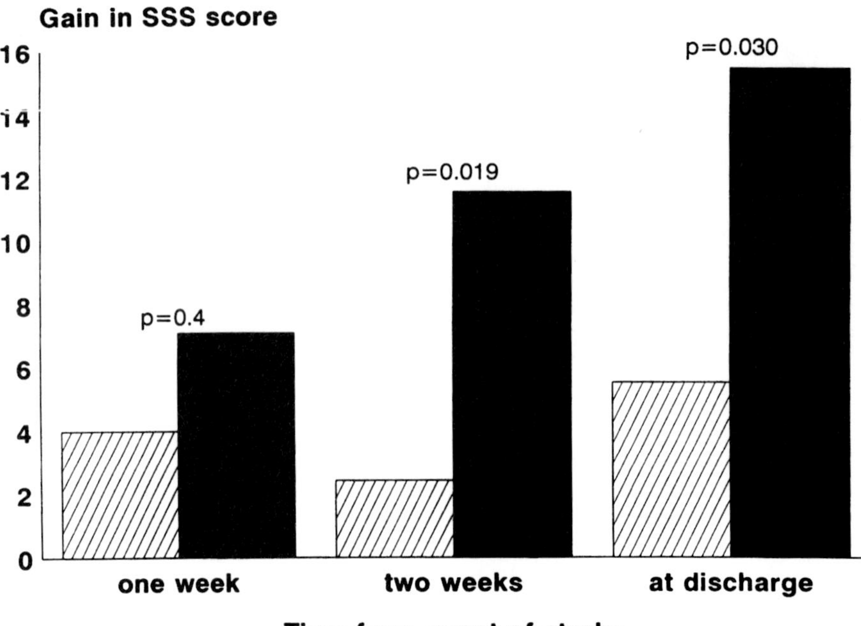

Figure 16-3. Gain in SSS score during rehabilitation in patients with and without reperfusion within the first week post-stroke.

reperfusion of the occluded area is in fact a major contributor to clinical improvement during rehabilitation and that lack of spontaneous reperfusion may worsen outcome.

The demonstration of a hyperperfused infarct by SPECT within the first week after the stroke should be considered as a favorable prognostic sign.

References

1. Olsen TS. Regional cerebral blood flow after occlusion of the middle cerebral artery. *Acta Neurol Scand* 1986;73:321–37.
2. Dalal PM, Shah PM, Sheth SC, Deshpande CK. Cerebral embolism: angiographic observations on spontaneous clot lysis. *Lancet* 1965;1:61–64.
3. Lassen NA. The luxury perfusion syndrome and its possible relation to acute metabolic acidosis localized within the brain. *Lancet* 1966;2:1113–15.
4. Jørgensen HS, Sperling B, Nakayama H, Raaschou HO, Olsen TS. Spontaneous reperfusion of cerebral infarcts in patients with acute stroke. Incidence, time course, and clinical outcome in the Copenhagen Stroke Study. *Arch Neurol* 1994;51:865–73.
5. Andersen AR. ^{99m}Tc-d,1-hexamethylene-propyleneamine oxime (^{99m}Tc-HMPAO): basic kinetic studies of a tracer of cerebral blood flow. *Cerebrovasc Brain Metab Rev* 1989; 1:288–318.

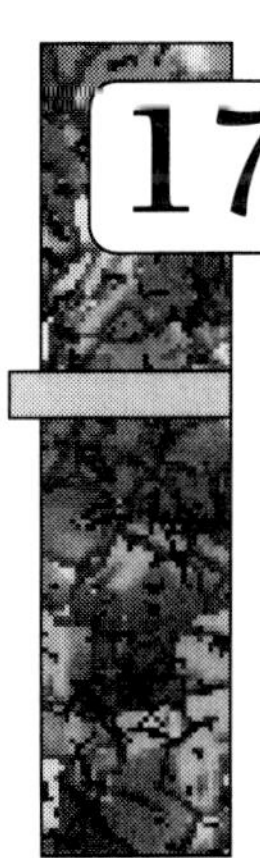

New NMR Methods in Rehabilitation Medicine and Research

James W. Prichard, M.D.

Introduction

In the last few years, nuclear magnetic resonance (NMR) technology has been developing so rapidly that it has opened the possibility of novel applications in a number of biomedical areas in which it has not figured prominently before. One of these is surely rehabilitation medicine. Extensive use of new NMR methods in rehabilitation research and practice is virtually mandated by the good match between the new methods and the current needs of the field. Rehabilitation specialists daily encounter clinical phenomena that are clearly important but are not well understood in biological terms. To the extent that this dispiriting barrier is due to lack of means for study of pathophysiological processes in the nervous system and in joints, NMR technology has much to offer.

This prediction is based on three inherent characteristics of NMR methods that together make them unique:

1. *Versatility.* About fifty different biological variables can be measured in clinical NMR machines in 1995. The number is growing rapidly and will quickly exceed one hundred; no one knows how much higher it will go. No other biomedical measurement technology can cover so wide a range in a single properly equipped instrument.

   Present capabilities include measurements in the central nervous system of anatomy, pathology, angiology, blood flow associated with function, and several aspects of normal and deranged biochemistry, including estimation of metabolic rates for glucose and oxygen. Dynamics of joint movement can be intimately assessed in individual subjects, and other aspects of joint function that have not yet been studied by NMR methods are within reach of them; the territory is rich and mostly unexplored.

2. *Noninvasiveness.* NMR measurements are among the most innocuous ones that can be made on living tissue. In theory, the magnetic fields they require

have no known deleterious effects, and none have been observed in well over a decade of experience in hundreds of centers. The hazards that do exist are well understood and minor compared to any measurement that uses ionizing radiation. Ferromagnetic objects must not be brought within several feet of NMR magnets, which can also erase the credit cards of the unwary. Pacemakers and ferromagnetic implants preclude some patients from having NMR examinations. Occasional anxious patients find the experience of lying in the magnet sufficiently claustrophobic to interfere with the test. All in all, however, invasiveness is so minor a consideration in making NMR measurements that it places little limitation on how they can be used.

3. *Cost-efficiency.* Upon hearing the claim that NMR methods are inherently cost-effective, the first reaction of most people in and out of medicine is incredulity. How can a $2,000,000 machine in a room that may cost another $1,000,000 if purpose-built be cost-effective? Indeed, at present, it is not. The claim is based on reasonable estimation of how NMR technology will affect biomedical economics in the future.

 Its unique combination of versatility and noninvasiveness ensures that the technology will improve accuracy of early diagnosis as physicians become adept at using it. Accurate early diagnosis means fewer and shorter hospitalizations. Every day a hospital stay is reduced is worth about $2,000 in advanced medical centers. Confident identification of patients who do not need hospitalization at all offers greater savings still, as do reduced consequences of inaccurate or delayed diagnosis. For these reasons, NMR diagnostic technology will achieve general recognition over the next few years as a tool essential for cost containment as well as for best medical care.

Rehabilitation medicine will benefit from these features of NMR technology in the same way that most other medical disciplines will, but it is also likely to benefit in ways special to itself. Without slighting the contribution of the rehabilitation community to society or disagreeing with its own leaders, one may note that the nation's rehabilitation engine runs on fuel containing more compassion, commitment, and common sense in deficit compensation than advanced medical science.

The reason is simple. A large proportion of rehabilitation problems involve joints and the nervous system, and repair processes are not well understood in either. Animal models are limited by large differences in species, age, and cause of disability, as well as by ethical constraints. For lack of observational capability, detailed study of repair processes in humans has not previously been possible.

It is now. NMR technology in mature form will be among the most powerful tools for extending knowledge of repair processes in the human nervous system, joints, and other tissues. It will never reveal everything one wants to know about them, and the things it can reveal will not come all at once. But NMR-based advances important for their daily work are sufficiently likely and imminent to engage the interest of nearly all rehabilitation specialists. Implementation of such interest need not be long delayed. The very general medical utility of NMR diagnosis ensures that state-of-the-art installations will soon be available to most rehabilitation research workers who wish to consider using them.

What follows is a brief account of some recent developments in the NMR world that are ready for clinical application and initial speculations about how they might be of use to the rehabilitation community. Several more general reviews of biomedical NMR technology are available (1–8).

Magnetic Resonance Imaging (MRI)

Most physicians are familiar with MRI as the emerging standard for diagnostic imaging. It is the process of making pictures of living tissue by use of the NMR signal from protons of tissue water. Like other soft tissues, the brain and spinal cord are 70–80% water, with a water proton concentration of about 110 M. The intensity of the water signal is sufficient to provide detailed information about human anatomical structure at the submillimeter level in an examination lasting only tens of minutes. Spatial resolution is determined by magnetic field strength and the size of the sample and is set exactly by the time that can be taken for data collection and by subject motion in that time. It is quite sufficient to create three-dimensional images that are already on the way to becoming a new standard for quantitative anatomical description of the living human brain and spinal cord.

Clinical images are most commonly made by a 1.5 Tesla instrument by placing the head or other region of interest at the center of the NMR magnet. While the subject lies quietly inside a cylindrical electronic coil, a small magnetic field gradient across the portion of the body being imaged is superimposed on the main fixed field of the magnet. Because of the gradient, water protons at different anatomical locations in the region of interest process at slightly different frequencies, which thus encode anatomy in a way that allows reconstruction of an image of the tissue by computer. Differences among the properties of water in different tissue compartments create contrast among the compartments. A variety of methods exist by which images can be optimized for definition of gray matter, white matter, cerebrospinal fluid, and other tissues. The low water content of calcified portions of bone causes them to appear as signal voids.

MRI is setting a new standard for quantitative study of normal anatomy in living humans, and it can define anatomical pathology at an unprecedented level of detail. Diseases processes with gross effects on tissue structure can be studied longitudinally as often as necessary, because repeated study by MRI is not limited by risk to the patient.

This kind of MRI has become "conventional" in the sense of being based on mature techniques that are available in most large medical centers. The advantages that conventional MRI offers to rehabilitation medicine include quantitative monitoring of the temporal course of atrophy and other abnormalities of deep structures unlimited by hazards from the examination.

Echoplanar Imaging (EPI)

Several techniques for collecting NMR data more efficiently have been devised (9). With fast acquisition, artifacts of cardiac, respiratory, and patient motion can be reduced or eliminated and the time resolution of NMR measurements greatly increased—to tens of milliseconds in some cases. Fast acquisition also facilitates getting as much diagnostic information as possible under constraints of patient tolerance and machine scheduling. The fastest technique is EPI (10), which uses rapid switching of magnetic gradients to increase the data collection rate. A two-dimensional image of 128 by 128 voxels can be acquired in less than 50 milliseconds by EPI.

EPI requires special gradient amplifiers that are not yet standard equipment on clinical imagers. However, its medical applications are so numerous that large medical centers are acquiring the capability as rapidly as they can. One of the most important applications is arrest of motion. Because motion artifacts can be very nearly eliminated, several kinds of NMR measurement that formerly were practical only in the head can be made in the thorax and abdomen as well. Cerebral blood flow changes and joint motion can be studied in real time by EPI. Both of these are clearly useful in rehabilitation medicine and research.

Magnetic Resonance Angiography (MRA)

MRIs made sensitive to the motion of blood water allow imaging of blood vessels without use of exogenous contrast agents. Arteries down to about 1 mm can be visualized in standard clinical machines. The cerebral venous system can be imaged with pulse sequences optimized for water motion at the slower rate that occurs in venous channels. Yet finer vessel structure can be detected by use of exogenous contrast agents such as gadolinium.

MRA requires no catheterization of vessels or injection of complex substances that can produce adverse reactions. It can be done in anyone who can enter a magnet, requires only a few minutes of additional acquisition time, and can be repeated as often as it is useful. When contrast enhancement is necessary, use of gadolinium can be justified more easily than that of x-ray contrast agents, which have more undesirable side effects. Cerebral blood flow measurements based on principles similar to MRA are being developed, and are likely to become practical enough for general use in the next few years.

In MRA, rehabilitation research has a potential marker for repair processes that would be of considerable value even if it were the only available NMR measurement. In fact, its biomedical value is greatly enhanced by its status as one member of a family of related techniques capable of making many other kinds of measurements.

Functional Magnetic Resonance Imaging (fMRI)

MRI pulse sequences sensitive to local changes in the concentration of deoxyhemoglobin can be used to detect changes in cerebral blood flow associated with local neural activity. Unlike oxyhemoglobin, deoxyhemoglobin is a paramagnetic substance that suppresses NMR signals from water molecules in its immediate vicinity. Because of this property, changes in deoxyhemoglobin concentration are detectable as local intensity changes on MRIs. Hence veins are darker than arteries.

Changes in deoxyhemoglobin concentration occur during local neural activity of sufficient intensity. Increased local neural activity is often followed by increased oxygen utilization to meet the extra energy demand. Cerebral blood flow and cerebral blood volume also rise, but to a degree which more than compensates the increase in oxygen uptake, so that the local concentration of deoxyhemoglobin actually falls. The consequent reduction of deoxyhemoglobin's paramagnetic effect results in a stronger local water signal. Signal intensity differences between MRI scans made at rest and those made during brain activation identify brain areas participating in the activity.

fMRI is not limited by use of radionuclides or other exogenous agents, and it does not require vascular catheterization. Cerebrovascular changes caused by any task that can be performed in the magnet bore can in principle be studied. Time resolution can be on a scale of seconds, since repetition of the measurement is not limited by hazard to the subject. Activation studies in the spinal cord have not yet been reported, but they are clearly possible. They may be especially useful for analysis of recovery processes after spinal cord trauma.

Neuroscience has had no previous opportunity to probe human neural function so deeply. Studies of brain activation by positron emission tomography (PET) provided a powerful new way to understand the human nervous system. The reach of such studies will be greatly extended by fMRI. Together, the two technologies will carry understanding of human brain function to a new level that only recently would have been thought fanciful. fMRI is likely to succeed PET measurements of cerebral blood flow with ^{15}O water as the principal method for studies of brain activation, because it has better time and space resolution and can be repeated at will. However, the exquisite sensitivity that allows PET to detect extremely dilute concentrations of labeled indicator can never be matched by any NMR technique relying on direct observation. Therefore, PET research on brain function will probably move toward exploitation of that sensitivity by placing new emphasis on specific ligand binding, a unique and already powerful capability that will grow in power as more ligands for identified receptors are developed.

Diffusion-Weighted Imaging (DWI)

When magnetic field gradients and pulse sequences are combined properly, MRI can measure the average diffusion rate of tissue water and express it as signal intensity in an image (11,12). Because the measurement is sensitive to motion of any kind, it is most valuable when made in machines that can use EPI to reduce effects of subject movement.

DWI detects ischemic brain tissue within minutes of onset in both experimental ischemia in animals (13,14) and in human stroke (15). The mechanism may be movement of water from extracellular to intracellular spaces as cells swell. Whatever its mechanism is, the phenomenon is of great clinical importance, because it can document brain ischemia or rule it out as soon as a patient with stroke syndrome arrives at a hospital. Conventional MRI does not reveal ischemic regions until they are several hours old, and x-ray tomographic scans remain normal still longer. Combined with conventional MRI, MRA, and other NMR measurements discussed below, DWI will become a mainstay of early specific diagnosis in patients presenting with stroke syndrome, and thereby facilitate prompt institution of appropriate therapy.

Another aspect of DWI capability that is potentially important for rehabilitation studies is emerging from experimental work on animals. Investigations undertaken for theoretical reasons have shown that DWI changes are caused by status epilepticus in rat brain (16) and can be largely reversed by phenobarbital (17). Preliminary evidence on less intense stimulation of the rat brain suggests that DWI sensitivity to brain activation may extend into the physiological domain under some conditions (unpublished observations). If that proves to be the case, a method for study of brain activation independently of blood flow changes may become available.

Magnetic Resonance Spectroscopy (MRS)

All of the measurements discussed previously are based on the NMR signal from the protons of water, which has a concentration of about 55 M in soft tissues. The great intensity of the signal from water overcomes the inherently low sensitivity of NMR to make possible the kinds of measurements described previously. For convenience, these are often referred to collectively as "MRI," while "MRS" is used to designate NMR study of much smaller signals from compounds other than water. Several dozen compounds can be detected in the living human nervous system by observation of ^{31}P, ^{13}C, ^{15}N, ^{17}O, and non-water ^{1}H. These signals are much weaker than the water proton signal, so that observing them takes longer, but acquisition times are within the range of biomedical utility for many compounds.

MRS information can be presented as chemical maps of the nervous system showing the anatomical distribution specific compounds, by procedures similar to the ones used in MRI, collectively known as spectroscopic imaging. In MRI, pictures of anatomy and the anatomical distribution of functional events are made from the water proton signal by coding space as frequency. The resonant frequency of water protons is changed in each of the three dimensions by placing a magnetic field gradient along each dimension, so that each spatial point has a unique frequency. A computer then constructs a picture in which the frequency differences are presented as anatomical ones. MRS signals can be acquired and processed the same way, but pictures made from them require more acquisition time and are far less detailed, because all MRS signals are much weaker than the one from water protons. Even so, technical advances are making rapid progress in presenting MRS data in readily interpretable forms similar to MRI (18,19).

The abundance of information available from MRS is indicated by the following partial list of compounds and derived biological variables that can be detected in the human brain in 1995.

^{1}H MRS: N-acetyl aspartate, glutamate, glutamine, γ-aminobutyric acid, glucose, creatine, several trimethylamines, and phenylalanine.

^{31}P MRS: phosphocreatine, adenosine triphosphate, inorganic phosphate, several phosphomono- and phosphodiesters, and intracellular pH (from the resonant frequency of inorganic phosphate).

^{13}C MRS: This nucleus is a stable (non-radioactive), magnetic isotope of carbon. Its signal is weaker than ^{31}P and much weaker than ^{1}H, and its abundance in nature is only 1.1% of all carbon (nearly 99% is ^{12}C, a non-magnetic nucleus that gives no NMR signal). Moreover, the only organic molecules in the brain that tumble freely enough to generate detectable NMR signals are small ones such as lactate, free amino acids, simple peptides, and some trimethylamines. Most brain lipids and proteins are complex macromolecules grouped in structures that constrain their motion to an extent that prevents detection of them in acquisition times practical for human work.

So what good is ^{13}C MRS for work on the human brain? Quite a lot. The same low abundance that places detection of most naturally occurring compounds out of practical reach allows remarkably powerful measurements to be made by observation of ^{13}C in metabolite pools labeled with it by feeding of ^{13}C-rich substrates (20). The ideal enrichment source for brain is glucose, metabolism of which meets nearly all of the adult organ's energy needs. In human stroke, feasibility of observing 3-^{13}C-lactate in the elevated lactate pool associated with the infarct has been demonstrated (21). Signals from glutamate, glutamine, and γ-aminobutyric acid are detectable in normal human brain after intravenous infusion of 1-^{13}C-glucose (22). This capability is entirely new. In its mature forms, it will probe the biochemistry of living human brain to a level of detail that cannot be approached by any other technology.

Still more powerful measurements based on ^{13}C labeling are possible by combined ^{1}H/^{13}C MRS. Detection of ^{1}H nuclei bonded to ^{13}C allows measurement of the latter *in vivo* at the much greater sensitivity of ^{1}H, thereby overcoming the signal-to-noise disadvantage of direct ^{13}C MRS (23). In the first example of its use to solve a neurobiological problem—as contrasted to demonstrating a new way of detecting phenomena already known to occur—this technique showed that lactate elevated by electroshock in rabbit brain is metabolically active, not trapped in non-metabolizing compartments (24). The same combined ^{1}H/^{13}C technique has been shown to be usable in human brain (25). With plausible assumptions about unmeasurable quantities, the data it provides can be analyzed by an appropriate metabolic model to yield rate estimates for brain consumption of glucose and oxygen (26,27). These methods are still at an early stage of development, but enough is known about them to create the expectation that they will mature into the most accurate and versatile ways of measuring metabolic rates in the human brain.

What Will NMR Methods Do for Rehabilitation Research?

The question is more novel than the methods themselves. The NMR measurements discussed above are so new, and so obviously powerful, that all wise neurobiologists are watching closely to see how and how much their own areas of research will be affected.

Most of the participants in the meeting from which this volume emerged—certainly the present author—were startled to realize for the first time how naturally emerging NMR methods seem to match the problem of modern rehabilitation research. The latter is much in need of objective means for (1) analyzing mechanisms of injury response and tissue repair in human brain, spinal cord, joints, and muscle, and (2) monitoring effectiveness of treatment on phenomena prerequisite for observable functional improvement. These phenomena need to be more thoroughly understood in humans than they ever can be from research on animal models alone, however extensive. NMR methods may well provide the necessary means, on a broad front.

The better part of a decade will be needed to test that idea thoroughly. The first step is to imagine specific ways in which research strategy might crystallize around it. A few possibilities are suggested below, accompanied by a petition for indulgence from a rehabilitation-naive author aware of traveling beyond the boundary of his personal expertise.

- "Conventional" MRI and MRA together will surely allow more thorough assessment of the extent of brain and spinal cord injury and the course of anatomical recovery from it than is possible by other diagnostic methods.
- MRI accelerated by EPI will document the three-dimensional anatomy of the living human nervous system in a degree of detail far beyond anything previously possible. By that much, anatomical aspects of brain and spinal cord injury and recovery critical for rehabilitation will be better known in each patient.
- DWI may facilitate early evaluation of rehabilitation potential by revealing the location and extent of tissue injury more prescisely than anatomical MRI.
- fMRI may be useful for early identification of candidates for intensive physical rehabilitation, by distinguishing those who can activate potentially compensatory regions from those who cannot.
- fMRI-detected activation of central structures by passive manipulation of limbs and electrical stimulation of peripheral nerves may provide unique assessment of the integrity of pathways essential for recovery, in the absence of the patient's ability to activate them voluntarily.
- Habituability by repeated activation of recovering tissue may be a sophisticated monitor of progress toward functionality; inability to habituate in a critical central structure may be the mark of a stalled recovery process.
- MRS is certain to document the biochemistry of injury response and tissue repair in human brain, spinal cord, and muscle after human stroke, trauma, and other afflictions. The information should substantially advance understanding of these processes, and it may provide early indicators of rehabilitation potential.
- Several NMR measurements may prove useful as surrogate end points for evaluation of rehabilitative surgery and other procedures; for example, DWI ought to detect populations of regenerating axon tips as they advance through a damaged region.

All of these possibilities are technically feasible. None is certain to be useful to rehabilitation specialists because of numerous empirical factors not yet evaluated. But the theory that basic advances come from basic research combined with the unique features of new NMR methods suggests that implementation of the latter in rehabilitation research and practice should be vigorously pursued.

References

1. Bottomley PA. Human in vivo NMR spectrocopy in diagnostic medicine: clinical tool or research probe. *Radiology* 1989;170:1–15.
2. Prichard JW, Brass LM. New horizons in neurology: new anatomical and functional imaging methods. *Ann Neurol* 1992;32:395–400.
3. Radda GK. Control, bioenergetics, and adaptation in health and disease: noninvasive biochemistry from nuclear magnetic resonance. *Faseb J* 1992;6(12):3032–38.
4. Stark DD, Bradley WG. *Magnetic resonance imaging.* St. Louis: Mosby Yearbook, Inc., 1991:2520.
5. Prichard JW, Rosen BR. Functional study of the brain by NMR. *J Cereb Blood Flow Metab* 1994;14:365–72.
6. Prichard JW. The NMR revolution in basic and clinical neuroscience. *Neuroscientist* 1995 (in press).
7. Prichard JW. Human brain spectroscopy: applications to normal function and neurological disease. In: Grant DM, Harris RK, Young IR (eds.). *Encyclopedia of NMR.* Chichester: John Wiley & Sons, 1995 (in press).
8. Prichard JW. Magnetic resonance spectroscopy of the brain: prospects for clinical application. In Young IR, Charles HC (eds.). *Magnetic resonance spectroscopy: clinical applications and techniques.* London: Martin Dunitz Ltd., 1995 (in press).
9. Frahm J, Gyngell ML, Hanicke W. Rapid scan techniques. In: Stark DD, Bradley WG (eds.). *Magnetic resonance imaging.* St. Louis: Mosby Yearbook, Inc., 1992:165–203.
10. Stehling MK, Turner R, Mansfield P. Echo-planar imaging: magnetic resonance imaging in a fraction of a second (review). *Science* 1991;254(5028):43–50.
11. LeBihan D, Turner R. Diffusion and perfusion. In: Stark DD, Bradley WG (eds.). *Magnetic resonance imaging.* St. Louis: Mosby Yearbook, Inc., 1992:335–71.
12. Moseley ME, Wendland MF, Kucharczyk J. Magnetic resonance imaging of perfusion and diffusion. *Topics in Magnetic Resonance Imaging* 1991;3:50–67.
13. Mintorovitch J, Moseley ME, Chileuitt L, Shimizu H, Cohen Y, Weinstein PR. Comparison of diffusion- and T2-weighted MRI for the early detection of cerebral ischemia and reperfusion in rats. *Magn Reson Med* 1991;18:39–50.
14. van Bruggen N, Cullen BM, King MD, Doran M, Williams SR, Gadian DG, Cremer JE. T2- and diffusion-weighted magnetic resonance imaging of a focal ischemic lesion in the rat brain. *Stroke* 1992;23:576–82.
15. Warach S, Chien D, Li W, Ronthal MB, Edelman RR. Fast magnetic resonance diffusion-weighted imaging of acute human stroke. *Neurology* 1992;42:1717–23.
16. Zhong J, Petroff OAC, Prichard JW, Gore JC. Changes in water diffusion and relaxation properties of rat cerebrum during status epilepticus. *Magn Reson Med* 1993;30:241–46.
17. Zhong J, Petroff OAC, Prichard JW, Gore JC. Barbiturate-reversible reduction of water diffusion coefficient in flurothyl-induced status epilepticus. *Magn Reson Med* 1993;33:253–56.
18. Brown TR. Practical applications of chemical shift imaging (review). *NMR in Biomedicine* 1992;5(5):238–43.
19. Alger JR, Symko SC, Bizzi A, Posse S, DesPres DJ, Armstrong MR. Absolute quantification of short TE brain ^{1}H-MR spectra and spectroscopic imaging data. *Journal of Computer Assisted Tomography* 1993;17(2):191–99.
20. Behar KL, Petroff OAC, Prichard JW, Alger JR, Shulman RG. Detection of metabolites in rabbit brain by ^{13}C-NMR spectroscopy following administration of [1-^{13}C] glucose. *Magn Reson Med* 1986;3:911–20.

21. Rothman DL, Howseman AM, Graham GD, et al. Localized proton NMR observation of [3-^{13}C] lactate in stroke after [1=^{13}C] glucose infusion. *Magn Reson Med* 1991; 21(2):302–307.

22. Gruetter R, Novotny EJ, Boulware SD, et al. Localized ^{13}C NMR spectroscopy in the human brain of amino acid labeling from D-[1-^{13}C] glucose. *J Neurochem* 1994; 63:1377–85.

23. Rothman DL, Behar KL, Hetherington HP, den Hollander JA, Bendall MR, Petroff OAC, Shulman RG. ^{1}H observed ^{13}C decoupled spectroscopic measurements of lactate and glutamate in the rat brain in vivo. *Proc Natl Acad Sci USA* 1985;82:1633–37.

24. Petroff OA, Novotny EJ, Avison M, Rothman DL, Alger JR, Ogino T, Shulman GI, Prichard JW. Cerebral lactate turnover after electroshock: in vivo measurements by ^{1}H/^{13}C magnetic resonance spectroscopy. *J Cereb Blood Flow Metab* 1992;12(6):1022–29.

25. Rothman DL, Novotny EJ, Shulman GI, et al. ^{1}H-[^{13}C] NMR measurements of [4-^{13}C] glutamate turnover in human brain. *Proc Natl Acad Sci USA* 1992;89:9603–9606.

26. Mason GF, Rothman DL, Behar KL, Shulman RG. NMR determination of the TCA cycle rate and alpha-ketoglutarate exchange rate in rat brain. *J Cereb Blood Flow Metab* 1992;12:434–47.

27. Mason GF, Gruetter R, Rothman DL, Behar KL, Shulman RG, Novotny EJ. Simultaneous determination of the rates of the TCA cycle, glucose utilization, a-ketoglutarate exchange, and glutamine synthesis in the human brain by NMR. *J Cereb Blood Flow Metab* 1995;15:12–25.